A FEW WORDS FROM THE CHAIR

A PATIENT SPEAKS TO DENTISTS

David Clow

Key visits

David Clow

Foreword by Lynn D. Carlisle, D.D.S.,
Author of In a *Spirit of Caring*

ISBN: 1-4392-1656-8
ISBN-13: 9781439216569

Visit www.amazon.com, www.fromthechair.com, or
www.booksurge.com to order additional copies.

*In memory of Norman Cousins,
and for every dedicated practitioner
of the art, science and business of dentistry.*

CONTENTS

FOREWORD BY
LYNN D. CARLISLE, D.D.S

Patients see things differently than dentists. Often, what is important to dentists is not important to patients. This seems like the hysterical discovery of the obvious, but dentists have a blind spot when it comes to seeing things from a patient's viewpoint.

They have a similar blind spot in their ability to communicate with patients. When asked to rate their ability to communicate with patients, 60% of physicians rated themselves in the top 10%. Dentists would probably have similar results.

David Clow's book *A Few Words from the Chair—A Patient Speaks to Dentists* does a great job of pointing out these blind spots and how dentists can eliminate them.

David contacted me after he read my book *In a Spirit of Caring* and Googled my Web site www.spiritofcaring.com. Both my book and Web site are about helping dentists build exceptional doctor/patient relationships.

David is a journalist/writer and was in the early stages of writing a book from a patient's viewpoint of the dentist's struggles with communicating with patients. Norman Cousins and Cousins' book *Anatomy of an Illness* influenced him. He wanted to write a similar book for dentists.

He asked me to review an early draft of this book and wondered if I thought there is a market for it. I did and I was very impressed. So were several other people - both dentists and non-dentists - who reviewed an early draft (see the Acknowledgements). This gave David the stimulus to go ahead and write *A Few Words from the Chair.*

A book about dentists from a patient's standpoint is long overdue.

Dentistry is either ignored or portrayed like an unwanted stepchild in the media, movies and TV. There are no national associations devoted to curing oral cancer, rampant caries, or advanced periodontal disease. None trumpets the wonders of restoring a person's smile, health and wellness as a result of a dentist's knowledge, care, skill and judgment. Grateful patients do not donate millions for a wing of a hospital devoted to dentistry.

Movies portray dentists as sadists or hapless nerds as in *Marathon Man, Little Shop of Horrors, The Dentist, 10, The In-Laws, Three Stooges, Waiting for Guffman, Wild Hogs* and *The Whole Nine Yards*. Cruel dentist jokes abound ("What are the six scariest words in the English language? 'The dentist will see you now.'" "It was worse than a root canal." "It was like going to the dentist.")

No books are written (glowing or critical) by patients relating their experience with their illnesses and dentistry like Norman Cousins' *Anatomy of an Illness* and *Human Options* did with medicine's treatment of him and his disease of ankylosing spondylitis. (These books were published in the late 1970's and 80's. They are still worth reading or re-reading.)

Until now.

This void is eliminated by David Clow's book.

In this brief, insightful book, Clow gives an outsider's perception of dentistry as a patient, writer and consultant. His perception hits a bull's eye when he writes that dentists are way off the mark when they ignore the person attached to the teeth and downplay the remarkable things they can do for a patient's health and appearance.

He thinks you spend too much time on gadgets and marketing at the expense of building caring relationships with patients.

He thinks you are capable of miracles.

He believes there is a great crisis in health care and an opportunity for you in preventing disease.

He also gives his ideas on why dentists sabotage themselves in the public and media's perception.

He asks enlightening questions about you and your dental practice.

Moreover, he gives you some ideas about what you can do to bridge the communications gap between you and your patients.

This book will help you see yourself and dentistry through a patient's eyes. Clow's perceptions will surprise you, open your eyes and help you understand your patients and what influences them in their choice of dentists. He relates why they make the decisions they do on accepting or rejecting your recommendations for dental treatment.

This book will help you be a better dentist.

Cousins' book led to a paradigm shift in how medicine viewed its relationships with patients. David Clow's book can do the same for dentistry.

Lynn D. Carlisle, D.D.S., Author, *In a Spirit of Caring, Understanding and Finding Meaning in the Doctor/Patient Relationship;* Editor and Publisher, www.spiritofcaring.com

ONE: OUR PRACTICE

Why this book?

Not long ago, I had a chance to give one of the best dentists in the country some comments about the ways in which he was marketing his services. This dentist owns one of the most prestigious and lucrative practices in the United States. It's not unusual for patients to fly halfway around the world to see him for a six-figure course of treatment, so his concern wasn't gaining more work or increasing his income. He wanted qualitative improvement. Although he had a beautiful office in a great location, dedicated staff and the finest equipment, he recognized that something was missing.

We visited together for over two hours, and he used part of the time to give me the talk he gives to prospective patients. He showed me slides of his beautiful clinic. He told me about his fastidious sterilization procedures and the purified water at every station. He took well-deserved satisfaction in the before-and-after shots of his work. His craftsmanship was breathtaking. Some cases started with severe damage. All of them ended beautifully. I felt deep admiration for his passion and his skill as he delved into the finer points of porcelain veneers. He makes his own, and he's an artist.

As he wrapped up his presentation, he looked to me with pride and waited for my feedback. He was right: something was indeed missing. "Doctor ___," I told him, "With all due respect, I don't care about anything you just said."

He wasn't pleased.

❖ ❖ ❖

Here's the problem: dentists and patients have extended interactions, but hardly any conversations. I assume the ones like this one with my dentist acquaintance are quite rare. That's too bad for us all, because I need your expertise, and you need to understand me better as well. Someone like you could be the most important health-care practitioner I know; people like me, typical dental patients, are the most important people in your professional life. When you and I don't communicate, we're both missing out.

With me, you have a chance to practice health care at a higher level, and for greater rewards, than you might ever have imagined. Speaking practically, you need more effective patient recruitment and better retention. You need to spend less time and money in areas that don't produce for you, and more where they deliver a return, so you need to invest as effectively as you possibly can at marketing, and more delivering paid services. Speaking at a higher level, you need the satisfaction of knowing that the work of your hands is making a difference, and that what you sow today is reaped in better lives for the people you treat. You want to enjoy the hours of your labor and you want to look back with deep satisfaction over what you accomplished. You want the respect of your professional community. You want to be appreciated by your patients while you're here and missed when you retire.

For all that, you need me.

What about me? Speaking practically, I need excellent health. I need pain-free, sound, strong teeth that permit me to eat the healthiest diet. I need to know the best mental well-being and the best physical fitness and the deepest emotional satisfaction a person can know. I need a trusted independent healthcare practitioner who delivers front-line prevention before my problems become serious, and even more—at a higher level—a chance to fulfill hopes and to find happiness of which I scarcely dare to dream. I need love, respect, joy and satisfaction in my life.

For all that, I need you.

Pretty ambitious, I know, and a lot for people to ask of each other. Does it surprise you that I should expect dentists to talk in these terms? It shouldn't. Your goals are the same as mine, and we can help each other to make them all real. For either of us, getting less than everything we hope for is foolish. Looking for less, and settling for too little, has had tragic consequences for every dentist and every patient in the nation. This unmet potential isn't a matter just of your income and my teeth. It underlies billions of dollars in poorly invested healthcare spending, millions of serious illnesses, and countless lives endured, but never truly fulfilled, by people who know neither how healthy they can be, nor the transformative possibilities of a smile.

Anatomy of an Illness

I'm not presumptuous enough to offer you technical advice. However, I don't hesitate to tell you that you that you're capable of miracles, and that I'm right to expect them from you. I'm very ambitious for us both in what we might accomplish together as great collaborators. Towards that end, I offer you this book, following one particular example: Norman Cousins' landmark book, *Anatomy of an Illness.*

If the title is unfamiliar to you, you might still know the case. Cousins' story originated almost fifty years ago, when the author, a highly regarded journalist and man of letters, came down with a form of arthritis that might have disabled or even killed him. This was the early 1960s, another era in medicine, a time when the patient and the doctor lived in different worlds. A serious illness placed the patient at the mercy not only of the illness itself, but also (and sometimes, even worse) of a medical establishment that tolerated the patient's presence, but relegated him or her to the passive and silent role of a coma victim. Hospitals were fearful places; physicians were remote, lofty experts; and patients were required to follow orders, period.

Over some informed objections, Cousins undertook to join his team of doctors as an active participant in his own healing, asking that his thoughts and feelings be heard, and even overriding their advice if he felt he saw a better way. He went home from the hospital. He quit taking heavy doses of aspirin. As part of his healing regimen, he took vitamin C by the gram and watched funny movies. He studied himself, learned the terminology, asked questions relentlessly, and didn't give up even when the experts told him he should. Against colossal odds, it worked.

His case was sometimes oversimplified or misinterpreted by critics. Cousins never said he saved his own life, nor that mainstream medicine was to be discarded. However, he did make clear that this new collaborative model was essential to his healing, and moreover, that every patient's contribution to their own version of this collaboration was essential in achieving the overall aims of any therapeutic intervention. Proving his own point, Cousins lived an active life far beyond what his diagnosis suggested was possible. The practice, business, and goals of medicine are all different today because of the experience he shared, first as the first layman ever to publish the lead article in *The New England Journal of Medicine*, and then in a best-selling book. His monument is the Cousins Center for Psychoneuroimmunology at UCLA, and his legacy, though he would be far too modest to claim it, is thousands of lives saved and improved by the ideas he helped to promote.

I had the honor to meet Norman Cousins when he taught at UCLA as an adjunct member of the faculty of medicine. (I also heard him share a stage for an evening with John Cleese of Monty Python's Flying Circus, discussing humor in medicine, and I can tell you, Cousins was a professor of humor too.) I got to tell him that his story was in my thoughts one night when I literally didn't know if I'd live until morning. On my wall, written in his tidy, precise script, is a quote from his book, the key lesson distilled from his experience and a call-to-action for healers and patients:

I have learned never to underestimate the capacity of the human mind and body to regenerate—even when the prospects seem most wretched.

Cousins' story of resilience and inquisitiveness inspired millions of readers, both laymen and medical professionals, and it shifted the doctor-patient relationship permanently from one of mutual misunderstanding to enthusiastic teamwork. That was a new paradigm back then. Today it helps keep people alive. His legacy is visible in every hospital and medical school in the nation that offers stress remediation and nutrition as standard practices, and that recognizes the patient as an essential member of the healing team, with the same ultimate aims in mind as the practitioner.

Norman Cousins was a hero. I'd like to make a tenth of the contribution he made to the betterment of the world. A hundredth.

The modern version of the Hippocratic Oath by Dr. Louis Lasagna includes a couple of lines that go right to the heart of why I am writing a book for your profession.

I will remember that there is art to medicine as well as science, and that warmth, sympathy, and understanding may outweigh the surgeon's knife or the chemist's drug.

I will not be ashamed to say "I know not," nor will I fail to call in my colleagues when the skills of another are needed for a patient's recovery.

I will prevent disease whenever I can, for prevention is preferable to cure.

I believe there is a great crisis in health care in the United States, and a great opportunity in prevention, and thus an essential contribution for you to make. I believe you are artists and healers with unique capabilities to make it. I believe there is a great deal we do not know about each other, and that it serves us both to talk.

❈ ❈ ❈

The gap

What an opportunity patients have!

Dentistry offers people so much they want and need. Why don't people get it? What would permit someone to have this resource available, and fail to use it? What would cause them to misunderstand it so thoroughly that they fear it more than they fear the consequences of *not* collaborating with a dentist?

There are gaps here, and like the gaps you work on in your practice, they're problems. The obvious one is between us, between dentist and patient. There's another between what I *really* need and what I *think* I need. Yet another divides what *you* think you do and what *I* think you do. And there's a serious one between the value most dentists have and the value they feel they can discuss.

It's especially frustrating because, after all, the interest is there on the patient side. I mentioned that more people are spending more money than ever on health care. I don't mean just mainstream medicine. Billions of dollars go every year towards alternative therapies and unconventional treatments. The wealthiest generation we've ever seen in America is ravenously consuming any credible product or service, and many incredible ones, to stay young and healthy. The key word there is "credible." Whether these vitamins and herbal remedies and prescription drugs and physical theories are actually effective is, of course, a different question. That goes for the mainstream medicine too, because it's highly debatable whether or not this medical colossus we've created delivers the most valuable care for the three hundred million people it's supposed to serve. So credibility and effectiveness may be separate. Indeed, they may conflict, and it's a safe bet that people are buying questionable and costly therapies not on proven merit, but on the hope against hope that they actually work (and if they do, the hope might well be the most potent aspect of the therapy).

And certainly, there are patients who try any alternative that will permit them a chance to stay out of conventional medicine, even when their lives are in danger.

Somehow, in the mix of these offerings, dentistry isn't where it belongs. Despite its credibility being beyond any doubt, this tidal wave of attention and money has flowed past the health care professionals whose services might deliver the greatest return of all. I'm not saying dentists are going broke, or that there are too many of you. Nevertheless, I'm struck again and again by the absence from both the patient side and the professional side of a big, factual, splendid declaration of the dental profession's real purposes and real significance, a statement so simple and truthful that nobody can deny it or get it wrong.

❖ ❖ ❖

I was surprised recently when I opened a best-selling anthology about healers and healing. It contained contributions by M.D.s and Ph.D.s, counselors, several different kinds of mainstream and alternative providers, but none—*none*—by dentists. Not a word. How is that possible? Were the editors suggesting that you don't have a place among such company, that you aren't "healers," while metaphysicians are? Is the dental profession suggesting that? Maybe the editors were asking, "What do dentists have to do with the health care crisis in America?" I'd hate to think that dentists are asking it too.

There's that gap again between the need and the solution. Frankly, I don't care who's responsible for it, but one way or another, it needs to be bridged. Whatever is standing in our way needs to be overcome by us both, together, because our goals here are the same and our effective collaboration is essential.

What an opportunity you have!

Great dentists perform wonders for their patients. Many of you hesitate to believe that, it seems, but I know you understand what I'm saying. I've spoken with dentists who were so moved by the effects of their own work they were almost reluctant to talk about it. They didn't want to seem full of themselves, or unprofessional,

I guess. From their modest perspective, they just fixed a problem. But the patient who rose from that chair, even after a brief course of treatment, was a different person, with a different outlook on life, with new hopes and possibilities, with courage and hope they'd never felt. That patient had been looking for that smile, or that relief from inexplicable pain, or the simple ability to eat comfortably, for their whole lives, and they found it in a matter of hours, in a place that once made them afraid, with a person they once avoided.

Miraculous, I'd say.

It's a humbling thing, I guess, to be told that you have miracles waiting to happen in your fingers, but please, don't argue with me about this. I'm not flattering you, and I'm not exaggerating. It's simply true. I need you to believe it every day. Your training and technology have never been better. My understanding of what great dentistry can do for me has never been greater. We've never needed each other more, nor ever have we been able to do so much practical good for one another. So if the billions of dollars patients are spending in pursuit of miracles aren't going at least in part to every dentist in the nation, we're squandering each other's potential.

What an opportunity we have!

I hope it's clear now why I was so frank with my friend the dentist. I meant no disrespect. My appreciation for his commitment and his skills was sincere then and it has only grown, but now, as then, I am desperate for our communication with each other to get past the fear and the constraints that make only for mutual misunderstanding.

I want our collaboration to reach that level where my highest hopes meet with the best of your abilities. That's why it's important for me to be as candid with you as I was with him. For your good and my own, I need you to think again about who dentists are, about what you do and why you do it. And I need to offer you some thoughts from the person in your chair.

❖ ❖ ❖

TWO: FOR WANT OF A NAIL

Idle hands

If you're looking for bad news, enter "U.S. health care crisis" on an Internet search engine. In seconds, you'll have links to over 20,000,000 articles to help keep you awake at night. They cover the costs of and lack of insurance. They talk about the millions of Americans who receive no preventive care and no basic maintenance for chronic conditions. They discuss Federal and state spending spiraling upward as the rates of diabetes, obesity, heart disease, cancer, and chronic illnesses rise as well; and meanwhile, life expectancy in the U.S. rises (still trailing 30 countries), raising the prospect of a sizable population living extended lives characterized by prolonged pain, illness, and dependency.(1)

Americans devote 15% of the mightiest economy in history to healthcare costs, $1.6 trillion a year—and that's an old figure–more than ever as a percentage of GNP and in dollars (2); and the great improvement that should have long since occurred for all this investment is yet to happen. In fact, things get worse with each passing year. As more people come to rely on it, there will only be more strain on a system that is, in many opinions, broken already.

The statistics on this issue will be obsolete the moment I commit them to paper, so I won't go into detail. You probably know the big picture better than I do anyway.

Still, I hope you're as perplexed as I am that you have to drill down through hundreds of articles before one of them mentions dentists or dentistry. Those that do mention them include them as afterthoughts, as a by-the-way after the daunting catalogue of seemingly more urgent emergencies. I couldn't find an expert or a commentator who mentions dentists in the context of the overall answer. Indeed, judging by the absence of dentistry from this coverage, it seems reasonable to say that most of the "expert" observers of this dire situation haven't recognized the mouth as the entry point of so many problems, and haven't thought of dentists as part of the solution.

Imagine a war being fought against an implacable enemy. Imagine that war taking a deadly toll, year after year, and endless money spent on it without resolution or even progress. Now imagine that the first line of defense against that enemy, possibly the best, most cost-effective and accessible weapon we have, isn't mobilized to fight.

Am I being overdramatic? The comparison isn't a stretch when we consider that in 2004, total medical expenditures for full- and part-year uninsured Americans was about $124 billion. That's more than the nation spent that year in Iraq and on anti-terror programs. A recent *Washington Post* story estimated that spending on health care in the United States could double by 2017, reaching $4.3 trillion and accounting for 19.5% of the nation's gross domestic product. (3)

Yes, it's a war. It's that important, and it's that expensive. We're fighting it with one hand behind our backs.

You see, there's another number worth considering here. There are over 250,000 dentists in the United States today, and even more hygienists, serving about 300,000,000 people. Those numbers have risen in an unbroken upward curve for over 30 years. Every year brings over 4,000 new students into our dental schools, and every year 4,000 new graduates take the first steps in their careers. The problem you face is that your numbers grow, but the resource you represent has yet to be effectively matched against the problem. This affects you twice. Like the rest of American taxpayers, you help to carry the ongoing and growing financial burden of this disconnect. As professionals with a contribution to make, the longer you're not directly involved, the longer the urgent need—and the business potential this represents for you—both go unmet.

There are some even bigger numbers to keep in mind. I don't think I can quantify them precisely; I doubt anyone could.

If nothing else about traumatic illnesses is good, at least they come with some urgency. Action is required. Help is mobilized. The statistics of epidemiology and costs for serious maladies are carefully kept. However, we can only guess at the magnitude of the slower, more benign degenerations of the body and the spirit that come with chronic pain or slow inflammation or compromises over diet or just too few smiles in a person's life. No one counts those cases, although they are indisputably real. They're just normal, just average. Whole lives are spent in such bad bargains with damaged mouths, with a smile hidden behind a lifted hand or even missing entirely, and those cases don't get counted. No one considers them to be emergencies. Nobody compiles these statistics, but

I suspect you've seen many patients like this. It has to be frustrating—how such a thing could be acceptable? How could someone so readily surrender eating well, freedom from pain and the laughter and joy that find expression in a glowing smile?

People give that up sometimes. Often, in truth. And it's a decision, not just something they permit. They decide to live with that slow, tolerable tragedy. They never know, or they learn to forget, what's absent from their lives when they don't feel fine, when they don't smile, and the missed opportunities and untaken chances for joy fade from their lives a little more and a little more until they disappear.

Maybe it's a good thing we don't know those statistics.

❖ ❖ ❖

Benjamin Franklin explained all of this in *Poor Richard's Almanac* back in the days when Paul Revere made dentures from hippopotamus ivory and scavengers pulled teeth from the dead on battlefields for sale to dentists.

For want of a nail, the shoe was lost.
For want of a shoe, the horse was lost.

For want of a horse, the rider was lost.
For want of a rider, the battle was lost.
For want of a battle, the kingdom was lost.
And all for the want of a horseshoe nail.

Would you call this an exaggeration? Please, think again, because this little tale has you written all over it. For want of a single tooth, how many illnesses start, how many joyful moments are sacrificed? For want of consistent dental care, how many diseases take hold in people, how many cases of heart problems or chronic inflammation begin, and how many lives are lost, or perhaps even worse, endured in a state of managed suffering? For want of dentists and patients understanding one another, for want of trust and transparency between us, for want of me being in your chair when you and I need each other, how many underutilized, undervalued, demoralized dentists are there; how many expensive, unproductive marketing efforts do you pay for that fail to help you build your practices; and how many billions of dollars are being spent year after year of your money and mine on illnesses that need not happen, need never become acute, and need not undermine the future for us all?

❖ ❖ ❖

The Inner Smile and the Duchenne Smile

You've seen the transcendent smile on the face of the Buddha. I find myself looking with awe at that smile when I see it in photos or on artworks in a museum, and I wonder, what kind of health, what kind of bliss, must be present inside of a person to express itself so profoundly on the outside?

Several traditions of eastern meditation include exercises designed to cultivate that smile. The people who use them have some practical physical as well as spiritual effects in mind; in fact, they don't separate the two at all. For millennia, Buddhists and Taoists have taught that smiling is literally good medicine, insuring longevity and good health by freeing the body from bad moods and their negative physical effects. Destructive emotions become constructive ones with a real smile.

A "real" smile—that's important to note. These people weren't fools. They could tell when a smile was just stitched on to someone's countenance, and when it arose from within and blossomed for the world to share. A smile can mask insincerity and bad intentions, and it's easy to be drawn in by it. However, they also felt that a smile is so powerful, that using it has to change the user before very long. Even someone putting one on as a mask becomes affected by it, and sooner or later, it does its work. It makes itself real, as the Buddhist master Thich Nhat Hanh explains. *"Sometimes your joy is the source of your smile,"* he says, *"and sometimes your smile can be the source of your joy."*

There's a meditation yoga practitioners use as a way to clean out negative energies from within their bodies before those bad thoughts become dangerous and toxic. They call it an "Inner Smile" exercise. They stand, breathe calmly and let themselves relax. Then they visualize a big glowing smile moving down through them from head to toe, touching and illuminating their organs and energy centers, the *chakras*. At every place, they pause, breathe, and let go of anything that troubles or upsets them, or just doesn't serve. (Try it sometime; it's a little like shining a flashlight into an attic room. You might be surprised at the junk you're keeping in there.) Moment by moment, breath by breath, the smile inside them moves along, lighting its way, leaving a better feeling, a more pleasant and hopeful one, than the one that was lodged here before. By end of the exercise, the smile that blooms on the outside has deep strong roots from within.

If this sounds a little unscientific, consider the work of the French anatomist Duchenne de Boulogne.

In the mid-19th century, his work on the physiology of the smile differentiated between a genuine smile that comes from a sincerely experienced emotion, and a fake one that is affected and displayed, but not felt inside. Even with his primitive equipment, Duchenne was able to demonstrate that they aren't the same. They employ different muscles, and because the real one employs muscles that are less subject to voluntary control, it's hard to manufacture.

Duchenne's successors named the real smile in his honor, and the fake one they called the Pan American smile, after the airline. Any business name could have served as well. The fake smile is that one you get at the customer service desk when the person smiling at you doesn't care that you're a customer and has no intention of providing you service. These modern researchers were able to go deeper than Duchenne had. They investigated the differences in brain activity and blood chemistry produced by both smiles—Cousins was getting at this when he watched funny movies from his sickbed–and there too they found were wide gaps in the empirical measurements. People who smile from inside really are healthier. Laughter heals. Inner joy, it seems, really is good for you.

Among the most interesting studies following Duchenne is one by Dacher Keltner and LeeAnne Harker at UC Berkeley. (4). They scrutinized photos taken of a high school senior class in 1960. About half were obvious Duchennes, the others obvious Pan Americans, all obeying some long-forgotten photographer's request to say "cheese." You could easily pick out which was which at the moment—who among these kids really felt their smiles, and who didn't.

What was really interesting was the adults these kids became. Their youthful smiles were early indicators of their later lives. The students were contacted at ages 27, 43 and 52, and asked, how is your marriage? Are you happy with your life? Thirty years after this early indication, the people who smiled genuinely were found more likely to be married and to have stayed married; to have greater feelings of well-being and stronger social bonds.

It was just a moment ago that I quoted the Buddhist master Thich Nhat Hanh, but I want to repeat what he said, now that we have examined a more clinical approach to the point he made. "Sometimes your joy is the source of your smile," he says, "and sometimes your smile can be the source of your joy." It's true. It changes how you feel. How you feel changes who you are. He continues, "If in our daily life we can smile, if we can be peaceful and happy, not only we, but everyone will profit from it. If we really know how to live, what better way to start the day than with a smile? Our smile affirms our awareness and determination to live in peace and joy. The source of a true smile is an awakened mind." (5)

If in our daily lives we can smile.

If.

That's a big if for a lot of people who don't feel healthy enough to smile, or entitled to smile at all. Peace, happiness, and everyone profiting...pretty high stakes if they don't feel they're so lucky.

I almost wish the clinicians had proved Master Thich wrong, because it's frustrating, isn't it, that such a seemingly small thing can resonate so long and so deeply, not only in one person's life, but in the lives of the people around him. Such a small thing can change the entire life you live.

A smile, that's all. If you have one. If you feel it.

Readers, please, say this. Embrace it. Keep this simple, profound truth close to you: you build healthy mouths. *You manufacture smiles.* That changes people, inside and outside. It changes minds and it changes bodies. It changes lives and families and futures.

Take a moment to think of everything that your abilities mean to me, to you, and to the world.

Now, tell me if you'd be one of the people who still ask what dentists have to do with the big health care picture in the United States.

❖ ❖ ❖

The r/evolution of dentistry

If you're just joining the dental profession, you have advantages in training and technology that none of your predecessors had. I suspect this is of limited comfort when your dental school tuition was stratospheric and the cost of opening a practice is higher than ever. That your predecessors are better known in your community than you are doesn't help.

If you're a veteran practitioner, you're managing a wave of technological acceleration and changing patient expectations that could, by themselves, be a full-time occupation. And the new dentist opening an office down the street isn't there to make things easier for you.

One of the early reviewers of this book suggested that the high level of professional courtesy among dentists would outweigh any sense of competition among them. Frankly, while I would expect some measure of courtesy to be there, I would also find it perfectly unsurprising to find an accompanying, and possibly greater, sense of competition. None of you is *not* in business. None of you is in business to fail. None of you is naïve about that.

In one way, though, the playing field is level for both the new and the veteran dentists, because most of you face the same chronic challenge: case acceptance. Training and equipment might matter in helping influence some patients to agree to an extended course of care, but if the dentist isn't personally credible, convincing and confidence-building, the training is moot and the equipment is just overhead, and that's as true for a longtime practitioner as it is for the new dentist in town. Mastering the equipment and keeping up with continuing education are comparatively simple. Getting patients to agree to ambitious, expensive dental work is a tougher task, made tougher still when there are plenty of other things a patient wants to do with several thousand dollars, and when it's still not clear to them what all that money and all that time spent in your chair is really buying. Any long-time dentist reading this knows the frustration of explaining a visionary treatment plan to a patient who really needs the work, and having that patient say, "Gee, I'd really rather spend the money on X." X is, well, you name it—a new car, a new boat, a flat-screen TV, season tickets to the Indians…one dentist I know never wants to hear the word "Mercedes" again, because patients of his have actually chosen to buy one instead of investing in their mouths. Maybe that's the problem. Those patients view dental work as a frill, and if you're going to buy a frill, the ones that don't involve drilling and needles have an advantage over those that do. (Expensive sports cars don't hurt when you get them. They only hurt when you're trying to get *rid* of them.)

And even if it's a sensible investment, like a house or a child's tuition, it seems crazy to you that they'd pay for almost any version of X before they'd pay for a healthy new mouth. You'd get a thirty-year mortgage and not a thirty-year mouth? You'd prepare financially for your kid's graduation, and not do all you can to live long enough to be there? It's obvious to *you* why that doesn't make sense, but these patients don't get it. And what's worse, they don't see the problem with valuing X over their own well-being. You know a healthy mouth is like a healthy heart or a healthy liver. They might think it's, well, just *pretty*, and if that's all they think it is, then there are plenty of other pretty things to buy, and plenty of less scrupulous people selling them.

There's an old joke that comes to mind when patients don't get the value of the therapy: how many psychiatrists does it take to change a light bulb? One — but the light bulb has to want to change.

We're talking about case acceptance, not just remedial care. Remedial care is where you fix me back up to my usual mediocrity and we forget each other. Case acceptance is where you and I meet to realize our potential together. But even the patients who need you the most don't necessarily want to change when they expect pain, embarrassment and inconvenience as the cost, not to mention the money. They're incorrect of course, but that's not what matters. You keep up with the technology and the improvements, but patients don't. We aren't aware of the comfort and ease of treatment you can now achieve for us. And you're up against some of the most indelible negative stereotypes any profession ever faced. Everyone from Lewis Grizzard to Steve Martin to Lawrence Olivier has memorably shredded dentists in print or in movies, telling us that the person in that ominous white smock is, at best, some sort of oblivious dweeb, and at worst, a sadist with a sick sense of humor. Dentists get nailed even when the complaint isn't about you: when a reviewer really, really disliked a Céline Dion song, he took it out on you: "What never ceases to amaze me is how the trite-est, most cliché-ridden music often takes an assembly-line of lauded music industry professionals to perfect... Sinking ships are what I imagine as 'My Heart Will Go On' plows onward of four-plus minutes…is it no wonder why I have such fears of going to the dentist?" Even National Public Radio got in the act, albeit unintentionally. They recently ran a series on distinctive sounds, and one of the sounds they featured was a dentist drill. From the infuriated calls and letters they got, you'd have thought they'd broadcast tapes of human torture.

You know that dental technology and practice have advanced past almost every objection the old stereotypes raise. You know that dentists can now rightly claim many once-frightening procedures to be fast and painless. You know you don't all play Céline Dion in the office (no show of hands, please, from those who do). But one funny line from an old Allen Sherman song—"And if you'll kindly stop those ghastly shrieks, I'm through!"—communicates more powerfully, and longer, than a hundred rational arguments.

Search for "dentist jokes" on the Web and you'll get this: "Anyone know the six most frightening words in the world? 'The dentist will see you now.'"

Not good. Older than vaudeville, I suspect, and about a century older than dentistry as you practice it. But you can't beat a memorable joke with information like my dentist acquaintance gave me that day about porcelain veneers and how he autoclaves his scalers. You need a better strategy, beyond the same fruitless tactics. You need to address the gray areas of communication, not just the facts. We, doctors and patients, need to build a better collaboration.

Norman Cousins started a revolution that helped to transform medicine, and we're all better off for it. Dentistry needs such a revolution.

❖ ❖ ❖

What is your practice?

Let me give you a somewhat exaggerated take from the patient's perspective of our first appointment.

I'm on time, and I'm nice to your staff and I haven't swiped any magazines. So far, so good. Then I sit in your chair and you ask me, what's the problem?

And I say: "I'm having trouble getting dates."

Not what you expected.

"Well," you say, "uh, that's not uncommon, ha… but…"

"I'm looking for career growth, too, but I'm doing lousy in job interviews."

"Well, nobody likes those, but—"

"I'd like to get some investment counseling too. Long-term financial strategy."

"Investments? Uh, excuse me, but I'm a den—"

"And generally I'm feeling kind of down. Not depressed exactly. More like just blue. You know. Lonely."

You're thinking, is this guy crazy? You're standing there in a white smock. You have equipment for bite-wing X-rays laid out a foot away. Financial counseling? Dating advice? *Hello?*

"Look," you finally say with some exasperation, "I'm a *dentist*. This is a dental practice. My diploma is right here!" And it says something like *Universitas Washingtonii in Regione Columbiana sita omnibus ad quos hae litterae peruerint salutem...*

And very patiently, I tell you, "It's in Latin."

"Well, of course–"

"I can't read Latin. And let's be honest: you probably can't either. So can you help me get dates and get a job and feel happy?"

You lose it. "You don't want a dentist, you want a magician!"

Exactly! We're saying the same thing. We're just saying it differently.

Let me give you my take on what you do. (That's wildly presumptuous, I know. Join me in a little wild presumption, just as an exercise.) Here's *my* definition of your practice: *your practice is any good effect of your work, direct or indirect, for which you can reasonably take a measure of credit.*

I hope that sounds like a lot. It requires us both to stop thinking about dentistry in terms of price, and to start thinking of it in terms of value, and the true worth—the meaning to me, the *effects*—of what you do. It begs a lot of important questions.

In a few words, what are you? Professional, expert, competent...I know you could keep answering with words like that. You'd be perfectly correct, and you wouldn't capture any more than what's obvious. And for our collaboration, obvious isn't working.

Are you repairman, mechanic, emergency technician, facilitator, counselor, confessor, visionary, partner, friend? I've heard all those terms applied by dentists to themselves, or by patients to dentists. They're a little less obvious than "professional" and "expert," but no less true. Some of them are more flattering than others (you'd hope the more flattering ones are the ones your patients share when they talk about you). And while you do have some influence over the things they say, your patients will still choose their own words to describe you. I'm guessing they won't describe you as "professional, expert, competent," though, because those are givens. Nobody's going to recommend your practice by saying, "I just found a *professional* dentist—and she's *competent!*" (Followed, no doubt by, "No more do-it-yourself extractions with a Vise-Grip for me!")

You'd like your patients to say the best things about you, and to be appreciated in the best possible ways by them. How do *you* see *them*? Are they teeth, mouths, caries, procedures, accounts, clients, receivables...? Be careful how you answer this. Your assumptions have a way of revealing themselves. I've been with dentists who casually mentioned the root canal at 10:30 to the receptionist, or the cleaning after lunch to the hygienist. I don't hold it against them that they're speaking office shorthand, but it does invite a little speculation—do they talk about me as "the crown at 3:30" or the "filling at four"?

There's a level of respect we need from each other. Let's go for the best. "Phenomenon" is what I'd like to hear said about you. "Superstar." "Artist." "Craftsman." Pick the one you like, and don't be modest, because it's entirely accurate—if you choose to make it so. It depends on you, and on how firmly you embrace that "good effect" definition of your practice. And if I'm the "filling at four," you're offering too little. Professional and competent are the least I want to expect. What I really want is for you to make me what happens when you're a genius.

❖ ❖ ❖

Let me ask you, what is your practice? Where is it? When is it? Who is it?

Answer these questions narrowly, and you'll give me what's on your business card—general practice, orthodontics, etc.; your address; your hours; and your name, D.D.S. or D.M.D. All of which tells me pretty much nothing. The "good effects" dentist, aiming a little higher, has more ambitious aspirations for us both: Here's how I define your practice: *Your practice is my mouth, my body, my physical well-being, my happiness, my career, my family, my dreams, my whole life.*

My whole life, that's what it is. That's how much you can affect me.

Where is it?

It's where I am, being that I'm your patient, so it's at my home, my work, and anywhere else I happen to be.

When is it?

It's 24/7, year-round, because that's when I'm the beneficiary of your skills, your goals, and your hopes for me.

And who is your practice?

It's us, you and me, and you and every other patient you serve.

Is all that impossible, excessive, unprofessional? Maybe. I suspect we're not going to see all that on your business card. But is it untrue? I don't think so. I think all that sums up very reasonably an optimal and realistic relationship between a great dentist and a great patient. You *do* have those effects. Your work *does* touch my life those ways. I wouldn't put up any billboards about it, at least not in that detail; but I'd urge you to consider the good you do, *all* the good you do, directly and afterwards, and to take a little credit for it. Take some responsibility for it too, as you ask yourself what your practice really is.

Again, this is your call. I'd speculate that those dentists who wish they'd done something else (There are lots of them, it seems, according to a survey I read about. I'll mention more about that later.), whose hopes got dimmed somewhere, are some of the same ones who confine themselves to the strict and narrow professional description of what they do, or think they do. After years of practicing professionally, expertly, and competently, they remained unaware of, or somehow unwilling to accept and embrace and savor, all the effects of the small miracles they make. And the excitement they felt when they started in dentistry faded. What a waste.

❦ ❦ ❦

It's a choice. The mindset you choose to define and invigorate your practice helps you find the joy in what you do. If you know all the effects of your work, and seek to deliver the best of the best, I don't know how you could get tired of it. Satisfaction like that could make you eager to come to work every day. Sharing that kind of commitment with your patients could make them eager to be part of your practice.

It might sound fluffy and highfalutin' to talk this way, and I know that dentists tend to think conservatively and scientifically. I'm glad you do. I'd say we're both being conservative here. The emotional and the scientific sides of dentistry are inseparable. The facts of what you do and the meanings of what you do are two aspects of the same real work that you perform every day. They both have everything to do with the marketing success of your practice and with your bottom line.

I don't think I'm presuming at all to remind you of all this, of things I'm certain are literally true, and that we both need to remember. It's a very rare profession whose miracles are so factually and routinely demonstrable; so much so, in fact, that the miracle workers themselves sometimes don't see them at all.

❖ ❖ ❖

Let's take a moment before we go on to talk about that word, "miracles."

One of my early reviewers for this book is a dear friend and a distinguished practitioner whose counsel I've valued since she was in dental school. She was concerned that the word comes with more hope, possibly false hopes, than any practitioner can responsibly offer.

Dental work doesn't make sad marriages or unfulfilling careers go away, she reminded me. It doesn't take off forty pounds and it doesn't restore eyesight. Fair enough. I offered in response that what it might do, though, is bring me to that seemingly improbable and perhaps forgotten tipping point, that toehold—just enough of a lift for me to start believing again in the changes I might actually be able to make for myself, my health, my present and my future. Some of those might be miraculous for me. She was willing to allow that. (She teaches dental students, by the way. This begins to explain why they love her.)

I appreciate her interest and yours in communicating with impeccable responsibility. Don't forget, though, what I might make of the opportunity you give me. If you've invested so much time and money in your work, and it doesn't include this kind of practical passion, and the simple acceptance of the great good you can do, you'll know it, and I'll know it. If it does, we'll both see the effects of it in your office and out of it—in your entire career and in my entire life.

Speaking as a member of your practice, I'm on your side here—I want you to make a lot of money, love every day, and take huge satisfaction from seeing the difference you make in the people you help. And I'm not settling for less than all the results I can get from a dentist practicing at the highest level, from someone who understands and pursues for me every good effect of excellent dental care.

❖ ❖ ❖

What *aren't* patients assuming about dentists?

Why did you go into dentistry? What have been your best moments in practice? Is it more satisfying for you now than it was when you began? Has being a dentist fulfilled all your hopes? Is it all you wanted it to be, or is something lacking? In doing my research for this little book, I was gratified to find that many dentists got into the field because they view it as creative, even as an art; that they see themselves as true healers and true teachers. Sadly, I also found that many others remain wedded, for better or worse, to the drill-fill-bill paradigm. The latter school of thought, no matter how well-intentioned, is part of the gap between many dentists and patients, and therefore part of the greater problem. If you are not fulfilling your highest aspirations as a dental professional, the problem isn't just your own. It's the problem of everyone who is avoiding your chair and missing the chance to be served by you.

Think about the things that you wish people took for granted about you and your practice. Each one of them would be a powerful selling point for new and repeat patients. If they were all true for every patient you treated, chances are you wouldn't need to spend a dime on marketing.

- Can you say truthfully that you know your patients personally? Would your patients say that you do?

- Do your patients hear from you beyond appointment reminders and perfunctory holiday greetings? Do you ever offer them information other than ideas strictly related to dental health?

- Do you keep your patients up to date on the technology in your office, so they understand not only why it's there, but what value you feel it has for their dental and overall health?

- Do you understand the secondary and tertiary effects of what you do, in your chair and beyond it, and do your patients know that you understand them?

- Do your patients feel a sense of personal empathy from you? Do they think of you as a healer? Do they trust you?
- Have you ever alerted your patients to a non-dental medical issue about which they needed to act? Would any of your patients ever say that you helped to save their lives?
- Do your patients know you love what you do, and why? Have you ever communicated to them the passion you feel for dentistry, and the satisfaction you feel from doing it superbly?
- Have you ever asked or been asked to give talks about dental care to gatherings outside your office? Who approaches you to do it? What do you say, and why? Who do you talk about, you or your patients?
- Are you "the" dentist, "a" dentist, or "my" dentist to your patients?

No matter whether you're starting out, or a long-time practitioner, "no" to any of these isn't good. The patients who experience dentists like that are probably the ones who don't see a dentist more than once a year, if that much. They're the ones who buy the Mercedes, but who don't invest ten minutes with a penny's worth of dental floss. They're the ones putting a small fortune away for their kid's education, but not doing the simple things they need to do so they're alive to attend the graduation ceremony.

They don't see this as a problem, even when they live, or don't live, with the effects.

❖ ❖ ❖

THREE: IMPOSSIBLE POSSIBILITIES

Your ideal practice

Someone took a poll recently asking dentists about the characteristics of an ideal practice. I have to say, the results struck me as disappointingly generic. Most of the criteria they listed, such as "interesting work," "team morale," "good management," "self-esteem" and so on, could have applied to just about any profession. Astronauts and caddies and sound technicians and the guys from UPS want interesting work, teamwork, good management and self-esteem. What was really surprising, though, was that none of the dentists in the poll emphasized *patients*. There was just one mention of them at all, in the context of a nutritionist's opportunities for advancement in a practice.

That was hard for me to understand. I can't imagine a practice mission statement not explicitly mentioning service to patients or pledging to deliver quality treatment to patients. It seems obvious, and as hackneyed as mission statements can be, the focus on patients should at least be mentioned, if for no other reason than simple business realism. No patients? No business. You can't practice dentistry without patients any more than they can have dentistry without you.

It seems equally obvious that anyone in an entrepreneurship like a dental practice would mention, above all else, the desire to secure the long-term loyalty of *great* patients, the patients willing to invest their time and money in having beautiful mouths and great health; the ones who'll refer their like-minded friends. Patients like that are highly desirable because they listen to your advice, spend their own money on you, and they do your marketing for you. Maybe it's so obvious that it seems acceptable to *imply* that patients are part of the work, but still, it's possible for a dentist to have interesting tasks and teamwork and self-esteem and all that, and go whole days without seeing a patient. Put a few days like that together, and what's implicit, but not actually purchasing your services, will be an explicit problem.

It's unfair, I know, to single out one survey and imply that it's indicative of the whole profession's attitude. Still, it crystallizes the issue, and any time you can learn from someone else's mistakes is better than any time you have to learn from your own. Any dentist in your territory who isn't aggressively dedicated to patient service, or who fails to communicate that commitment to his or her patients, is doing you a favor. Professional courtesy? Maybe. But there isn't a dentist reading this who ever sent a patient back to his old dentist out of professional courtesy when the patient was looking for someone better.

You're in a competition with so many practitioners, I'd suggest that you don't have much choice except to be businesslike, ambitious, and innovative in just about every area of your practice over and above being trustworthy and honest. With a quarter of a million dentists out there, with several of you working shoulder-to-shoulder in many places, you're working every day to distinguish yourself. You're also up against the entrenched negative thinking of your prospective patients, who don't necessarily want to want you, and who, even when they need you, prefer to spend the time and money anywhere else but under your care.

And you might face an even more powerful adversary in your own assumptions. If you're one of the dentists like the ones in the survey, who, even with the best intentions, just implies what needs to be communicated to patients explicitly and repeatedly, walk to the mirror and take a look at your most effective competition. The dentist you see is, putting it politely, the one who's cleaning your clock.

❖ ❖ ❖

Dr. Lynn Carlisle is the dentist/writer who told me about the poll I mentioned earlier. There's a discussion about another telling poll in his remarkable book *In a Spirit of Caring*. He quoted a survey in *Dental Economics* magazine of over 500 practitioners who were asked, "If you had to do it over, would you become a dentist again?" It seems that about 250 respondents answered no. I don't expect you to be any happier in your work day after day than I am in mine, but then again, if you think that number is discouraging for a dentist to hear, imagine being a patient and knowing there's a one-in-two chance that the person holding that whining drill is burnt out, bored, and would rather be golfing.

How therapeutic might it be for us both to share a real collaboration in which I'm your reliable repeat patient, with high aspirations and the willingness to finance them, and you're my counselor, my mentor, and the artist who can help me realize my fondest hopes?

How productive might it be if we understood completely every contribution we could make to each other's lives?

❖ ❖ ❖

I'd love to ask these questions of M.D.s, but the hope that they'd ever be able to answer in the affirmative seems pretty unrealistic. I see my doctor annually for maybe half an hour. I say "my" doctor, but there's no possibility really that they're "mine," and the next annual visit might be with a different doctor if the HMO I'm with this year says so. If that doctor is holding the wrong chart, the first question he asks might be about my morning sickness, while the lady in the next room is being asked about her prostate. That's life when you're a patient in the modern medical system. You feel like a number.

There's a lot more reason to hope for you being "my" dentist, and "my" front-line healthcare ally. My visits with you probably are more frequent than they are with my doctor. We spend more time together in an average appointment that I ever do with an M.D., and I'm probably more comfortable with you in your office than I am in an impersonal examination room, where I've had my blood pressure taken by the aide who didn't introduce herself, and where according to some universal medical policy they have the air conditioning turned down to meat-storage temperature while I'm shivering in a paper gown waiting for a highly unpleasant exam, that, ahem, doesn't involve eye contact. None of my many doctors has ever given me a simple full-mouth exam. It's entirely reasonable to think that you'd catch the signals of some incipient problem, even a life-threatening one, before a physician does, or more important, after a physician fails to. It's just as likely that you'll save my life as it is that they will.

Dentists are independents, the last practitioners whose allegiances are local and personal, and I assume confidently that what you tell me comes from you, not your consortium or your PPO or some distant interest tying your hands and compromising my relationship with you. Think of it: to the doctor assigned to me by my provider, I'm patient 245-8L, but you recognize me every time I see you. Your staff knows me. You don't have to call the central administrator or the main office or the United Nations to propose a treatment plan. You can talk with *me* about it!

I don't take any of this for granted, but I wonder sometimes if dentists do. If patients are assumed, then perhaps a lot of the good you do patients is assumed as well. I'm guessing that much of the value you deliver might not factor into the overall ways in which you measure your performance, or into the ways you communicate your importance, or into the satisfaction you derive from doing your jobs well.

We both need that to change.

✤ ✤ ✤

Ms. Johnson never smiles

As scientists, you've been trained to hold anecdotal evidence at arm's length. As a patient, I'm likely to base my opinion of you solely on anecdotes. I won't be so diligent as to seek statistical significance in polling friends and acquaintances to find a good dentist. If someone I trust gives me a recommendation, just one story might be enough.

Consider what a story like this tells me.

Ms. Johnson is a schoolteacher. She's young, in her third year out of grad school. She loves kids. She's known all her life that she wanted to teach. After years of focused training, two degrees, internships and a dozen interviews, she got her dream job teaching at an elementary school in Kansas City. She couldn't love her twenty-seven second graders any more if they were her own.

The problem is, they don't love her. They get quiet when she's around them in the schoolyard. They whisper. It's been this way since the first day. Beset by doubts and anguish, she feels her old confidence badly shaken, and she hurts. She goes home some nights and weeps.

She's afraid to discuss this with her principal or her colleagues. She drives forty miles to talk with a psychologist because she doesn't want people in her neighborhood to know that the teacher needs counseling. It's affecting her personal life. It threatens her relationship with a man who wants to marry her, but whom she pushes away, fearing that she's a failure, that she's made a terrible mistake and that her lifelong hope for a career doing what she loves won't happen. She's unhappy in her job, unhappy in her life, unhappy with her future. Her doctor has prescribed antidepressants. Ms. Johnson hasn't opened the bottle yet because she hates the idea of taking "happy pills," but she feels the sadness coiling tighter and tighter around her like a big cold snake.

One day she overhears two of her second-graders talking, and one of them says, "Ms. Johnson never smiles."

Of course she doesn't. Her family never valued beautiful teeth. They didn't have a regular dentist. She got accustomed long ago to laughing behind her hand, and to catching a grin before it got big enough to embarrass her. Money isn't the issue—she gladly spends her own money on paper and crayons for her kids, and less gladly, a hundred dollars an hour on talk therapy. But dentists, to her, are a just a last resort to fix an intolerable toothache. She doesn't go until it hurts, a lot. Dentists? Happiness? No connection.

But—three weeks after she hears "Ms. Johnson never smiles," her whole life is different. Her kids are head-over-heels crazy about her. Their parents want to meet her. Her principal notices the change. Ms. Johnson washed the happy pills down the sink, and the therapist she was seeing has been politely dismissed. Her boyfriend wants to propose.

You know what I'm going to say: Ms. Johnson went to a dentist and bought a smile. Speaking with more statistical accuracy, she went to a dentist and bought a million of them, and she's been handing them out by the bagful to her delighted kids. A seven-year-old woke her up in a way that the entire dental profession hadn't ever managed to. She'd looked for months for the key to her problem, and she found it in six hours in the last place she'd thought to look.

Speaking of tipping points, right?

A dentist told me that story. He didn't volunteer it. I had to ask repeatedly for him to go beyond the details about the procedure he'd performed, and to talk about what he'd really achieved for her. He spoke of the change in her life as though it wasn't really his doing. I guess it was admirably modest of him to decline credit for this, but then again, something happened here, and just as a snowball starts small somewhere before it gets big, credit for Ms. Johnson and all the other Ms. Johnsons you've met belongs to someone.

There's that choice again, the one between that literal, narrow practice mission, and the true effects of the practice. I guess my dentist acquaintance felt it would be irresponsible for him to presume too much about what he did. I suggested it was irresponsible for him to presume too little, because he might treat this Ms. Johnson as an anomaly and never try to make another one. The individual version of the effects would change patient-to-patient, yes, but this dentist's ability to *start* those effects would be the same. This dentist might very responsibly, very professionally, commit himself to making something wonderful happen for every patient he sees. He can keep that commitment. I asked him to believe just that much.

I want *my* dentist to understand effects like this. I'll pick one dentist over another one, and certainly a dentist over any other therapeutic provider, if they know they can have effects like this for me.

❖ ❖ ❖

Another joke comes to mind here: a guy loses his contact lens. He spends an hour looking for it on his hands and knees in the living room, and his wife finally asks, "What are you doing in here? You lost it in the kitchen." And he says, "I know, but the light is better in here."

People like Ms. Johnson and me look for solutions where we think we'll find them, even when they aren't really there. We might waste years, not to mention lots of money, taking happy pills, seeking fixes that are simply inappropriate to the real problem because someone—that Mercedes salesman, maybe—has encouraged us to look in the living room first, and because nobody is there to tell us that the problem really is in the kitchen. You've seen examples of this from the most innocuous cases to the most grave ones. Dentists have told me just how serious that error can become when a patient suffering from years of chronic head and neck pain has undergone surgery and prolonged medication and acupuncture and even psychiatric counseling, and finally, on the brink of suicide, sees a dentist and gets told on the first visit that they have a TMJ problem.

What if they'd missed that appointment?

Here's a variation on that joke: a woman spends years despairing about ever finding fulfillment in her life. She looks for it in the wrong places, in unproductive places, and, as the desperation mounts, she looks in dangerous, unhealthy places, and nothing works. She never has that instant of providence and insight about what she needs. No second-grader enlightens her. She sacrifices a career and a relationship. She blames herself, bad luck, everything but the real problem because she's sure that something so banal and ordinary as that—*teeth*, for God's sake—can't possibly make any difference. Finally, she gives up. And where she goes after that, well, it's only bad.

It's preposterous to think that a dentist could make such a difference in someone's life. *It's also completely true.*

I'm asking you to quit being modest about what you really achieve. I need to know that you know this about yourself and what you do, and to embrace that understanding in your practice as surely as you do any other irreplaceable asset you have. Ms. Johnson's story is the story of a thousand people in your neighborhood. They need what she needed, and you can help them, but not until you accept and share this knowledge. Until your prospective patients know what change a dentist can help them make, they'll still be looking, but not with you. They'll spend years searching in the wrong place for what's missing in their lives. Maybe they'll just give up looking at all.

That's the joke.

No, it's not funny. It's just terribly sad and it's all too normal for millions of patients, and for dentists, it's the success that doesn't happen.

By the way, the dentist was invited to Ms. Johnson's wedding. Several of the people closest to the bride understood what happened to her, and the difference that her dentist made. Word got around while the bride was smiling radiantly for the wedding photos. That Monday, the dentist had seven new patients.

❖ ❖ ❖

FOUR: FRAMING

Irrational economics

Adam Smith, the 18th century Scottish philosopher, is commonly credited with founding modern economics. I'd offer that he's the founder of modern dentistry as well.

Smith's great legacy is the idea that in a free market, people like me make rational decisions in their own self-interest. Inevitably, we, in making those decisions, also make things better for the society around each of us, because we're all rational, and all of us acting rationally create wealth for ourselves and for the society as a whole.

This idea, one of the central tenets of modern business theory, is known as the "Invisible Hand." Speaking of jokes, that one's a howler.

It's a leap, to say the least, to say that all my decisions are rational. On any given day, it's a leap to say that *any* of them are rational. If you look at the Internet Bubble, the Housing Bubble, stock market dips and jumps, most candidates for public office, or most prime-time television and Hollywood movies budgeted at $100 million, you start wondering if anyone making decisions in these situations could find the world "rational" in a dictionary.

And then, of course, there's the patient sitting in your chair.

Sure, this patient is perfectly rational. He sits there as you describe the overall effects of an ambitious course of treatment: better comfort. Better nutrition. Better health. Improved appearance. Uplifted morale. You've made this case quite rationally a hundred times, I know. You have before-and-after photos to help make your case. And the patient hears every point without arguing. When you're done talking, they say that you're entirely correct, but what they really have in mind for that ten thousand dollars is making a down payment on a new car. A Mercedes. Red with white upholstery. It'll make their whole lives better, they're sure.

So much for rational.

Okay, it's too much to give Adam Smith credit for modern dentistry, but we have to acknowledge his influence on modern dental marketing. The idea that the patient is thinking rationally is still the basis for most doctor-patient communications, it would seem; and that assumption is the source of a whole lot of wasted time and money, and of the frustration dentists feel when they offer dramatically better health and happiness to a patient, and the patient still says no. And it's not that the patient doesn't want health and happiness. It's that to the patient, that white upholstery *is* health and happiness, or more of it, at least, than what you offer.

Is that rational? If people were rational, nobody would smoke, nobody would have bought Yahoo! at $120 per share, and no one would think that a certain brand of beer makes them more attractive to women. Even better, we'd all be regular patients for our trusted dentists, there might not be any national health care crisis, and you'd never have to spend a dime on marketing.

Thanks, Adam Smith. You're fired.

❖ ❖ ❖

You and I, dentist and patient, enjoy our most fruitful collaboration in the realm of the irrational. Yes, the foundation for our relationship is the precise and very rational engineering you're paid for, but the best results from it, the purest satisfactions, are subjective and irrational and impossible to measure strictly by price. Your worth exceeds your bill to me, if you're good. I don't mean proficient. Proficient is the least I expect from anyone with a modern dental education. I mean *good*—good for what you intend for me, good in how you invest yourself. Good is a gift. It's irrational. It's genuine. It comes in many forms, some more valuable than others, but it's real. While the dentist was selling proficient, that car salesman was selling good. As your patient, I need you to include that way of thinking in what you do.

I understand if your instincts are all against this. The world is full of hucksters and second-story men selling big red cars. Dentistry is better than that, and you're better than that. You don't need to compromise the profession or yourself to use this idea. It's the difference between adequate and completely successful for our practice together. For me, it's what separates the adequate dentist from the great one.

❖ ❖ ❖

Our mutual values

Not all dental practitioners call themselves "holistic," and some might disdain the term because of whatever baggage or other comes with it. Fair enough; frankly, I think holistic means just about anything, and so it means just about nothing.

But whether you're holistic or not, I'm a whole. Until the day I can drop my teeth off at your office and pick them up later—which is never, I hope—then you're going to have to deal with all of me.

Likewise, I'll make my decision on choosing or keeping you as my dentist based on all of you, and probably not principally on your skills. I'm nobody to judge one dentist versus another, or one dental school against another one. I certainly don't want to do some kind of comprehensive survey to find you. I might call the famous 800 number, but then again, I'm guessing that all you need to be part of that registry is a license, so it doesn't tell me much. Ads from dentists come in the mail, and I see billboards and bench ads. Those don't tell me anything either.

The usual menu of media is changing very rapidly, and in ways you can't control. The Web makes it possible for anyone like me who moves to a new neighborhood to find public comments about every dentist in the Zip Code. What patients say there has to be taken with a grain of salt, of course, but I'll look very closely at a review from a patient who had a very good experience, or a very bad one, in picking a new dentist.

I'll probably find you by asking friends like me, in my neighborhood, but more important, with needs and interests like my own. If I hear good things, that could be enough to make me call. You might be surprised by what counts as "good things." Very likely they fall outside the services for which you get paid.

You're a dentist and I'm a patient, but those titles mean next to nothing in predicting the success of our collaboration. We're people, and this very specific reason for us coming together doesn't limit our interaction. It only starts it. Most of the rest of our contact is much more ambiguous. Dentists make impressions. It's a revealing pun, isn't it, that in your world that means one thing, while in mine, it means about a dozen other things. And we're both right. If I'm careless about being on time, if I'm unpleasant to your staff, if I swipe your magazines or take forever to pay my bill, I'm a patient second, and a pain in the neck first—a highly negative impression. If I recommend you to a friend, it'll be in similarly imprecise terms: she's "very pleasant," he's "like a friend," and so on. I'll say how impressed I was.

All of those ambiguities fall outside the hard conditions of our doctor-patient contract, and all of them matter. So you're never dealing with a "patient" any more than you're treating a molar in isolation from the rest of me. You're dealing with a whole person, mind and body, spirit and psyche. (Take a look sometime at a Weblog about the dentists in your area and see what people say. They'll find significance in things and attitudes you might not even notice, and they'll make ruthless judgments, pro and con, based on those.)

And you aren't a "dentist"; you're a whole person practicing dentistry, and if your hopes and dreams aren't part of that practice, every day, maybe they should be. Believe me, we'll know it very quickly if we don't inspire each other. If that feeling is missing, we don't have much of a future together, and we'll have to face the expense and inconvenience of replacing each other.

For want of a nail, right? You and I value the same things. You and I are each other's nails.

We need common ground, and we need it now. Every day that I permit my misunderstanding of what you do to keep me away from your chair is a wasted opportunity. Every mistaken assumption that separates us damages my possibilities and yours.

Among the many synonyms I find in my thesaurus for "impression" are "conjecture," "suspicion," and "guess."

They're all useless to me when I'm trying to make good decisions about my health and happiness. I'm seeking better impressions: my thesaurus also lists "confidence," "reliance," and "acceptance." Even "faith."

Good qualities. Give me those as readily as you give me the science and the engineering. Let me impress you with my eagerness for your best and wisest counsel, your skills, your experience and your caring. If we both make those impressions, we have a partnership. Put your heart into your hands for me. I'll put my hopes into your chair—punctually—for you.

❖ ❖ ❖

My frame and your frame

I have this wild fantasy: it's my first appointment with a dentist. The office asks me to show up half an hour early, and I go expecting to cool my heels reading about the 2004 Red Sox in an ancient issue of *Sports Illustrated*. Instead the dentist herself, or someone from her staff, greets me on time, asks me into a private office, and invites me to sit at a table. There's no equipment, no X-ray machine. It's just us. And this person, to my complete surprise, wants to know me. She smiles, looks me in the eyes, asks me questions and takes notes. She asks about my diet and my habits and my job and my exercise routine. She gets my whole history of prior dental care. She smiles and looks for me to respond in kind.

I get the strange feeling that I'm being observed very closely, not intrusively, but with kindness and real interest. I relax and open up to her. We're sharing pure impressions here, not much clinical information, but I understand that what is being communicated has value for my long-term health and to her long-term business relationship with me.

Besides, she's *nice*, and I appreciate that.

There's more going on here than I realize. I might think I'm hiding a great deal from this dentist because it embarrasses me or because it just doesn't occur to me that she's the person to deal with it, but she sees it anyway.

Did you ever read the Sherlock Holmes stories by Arthur Conan Doyle? The first time Holmes meets his friend Dr. John Watson in *A Study in Scarlet,* he startles Watson with what he sees:

"Dr. Watson, Mr. Sherlock Holmes," said Stamford, introducing us.

"How are you?" he said cordially, gripping my hand with a strength for which I should hardly have given him credit. "You have been in Afghanistan, I perceive."

"How on earth did you know that?" I asked in astonishment.

"Never mind," said he, chuckling to himself. "The question now is about haemoglobin. No doubt you see the significance of this discovery of mine?"

Your first examination of my mouth tells you a great deal of my life story. You can tell if I smile a lot or if I don't. You know if I'm a smoker. You might be able to tell how long I've been smoking, and how heavily. You can see signs of bruxism. You know if I eat a lot of junk food.

We've been discussing smiling and cosmetic dentistry a lot, but this exam you do gets down into some serious systemic health issues. You might see signs of diabetes or cancer. You might see inflammation and early warnings of heart disease. My mouth must reveal signs of chronic stress to you—compound that with the gingivitis, and the expression "heart attack waiting to happen" isn't just some one-liner. You have one sitting in your chair.

If there's an accurate biography of me, you're looking at it. My life story is written right there for you when I open my mouth. Between that and a few simple questions you might conclude very quickly that my job has me worried, my marriage isn't great, my self-image is bad...just as Holmes read Watson, you're observing clues about me that may well create the basis for our long-term relationship. You're seeing me below the surface, even seeing me as I fear to see myself, or just don't know how to.

For a mechanic, this might be out of the scope of practice. But for the dentist like this hypothetical one who's collecting very important data from me just by talking, the one who can really work there, the part below the surface is a very fruitful place. You and I can collaborate there very effectively if we change each other's frame.

A *frame*: it's an idea. It's the perspective I take, the boundary within which I live. My frame—frame of reference, my point of view, my *status quo*, if you like— might make it normal and acceptable for me, as it was for our friend Ms. Johnson, to live with a mouth I want to hide. My frame, particularly if I've lived with it for years, is where I look for answers and solutions. It's where the light is better for me. It might be completely foolish of me to believe it, but there it is. Within my frame, normal is a smile I hide, and hiding my smile is normal.

You might not think it's your job to help me *reframe* my thinking. After all, you aren't a counselor or a relationship coach, right?

But you want to sell me a comprehensive treatment plan. You want to give me that glowing smile you know you can make for me. So you need to reframe *my* thinking. You'll need to in order to get me emotionally invested in implants and veneers and whatever else is part of this course of treatment you want me to buy. If you don't, I'll stick with what's normal, thank you, and if normal is not smiling and living with moderate discomfort, maybe I'll use that ten thousand dollars on an investment that thrills and gratifies me.

Did I mention the Mercedes I just bought? I'll show it to you when they're done fixing it. Again.

That's ten grand that didn't go to your practice, and that was, in the end, probably a pretty unwise investment for me. (Funny thing about the smile you get from a new car; it goes away around the third time you have to take the car back to the dealer.)

I wanted a smile. But I bought it my way, inside my frame. The ads and the car salesman knew just how to communicate with me. I willingly let them influence my decision. Will I permit that radical a change in my life from someone who communicates in clinical, literal terms and jargon?

You want me to make a genuine, lasting smile part of my life? That means I, with your help, need to change my whole frame, my whole status quo. Okay. We'll break my frame wide open. I'll let you change the face I see in the mirror. But if I do, I'll be letting you perform some pretty radical alterations to my most fundamental assumptions about myself, and this goes way beyond teeth. You'll be changing me deeply and profoundly, heart and soul. If *your* frame, if your assumptions and your ambitions and your status quo aren't up to that task—if all you want to be is a mechanic—then no… no thanks.

Just a cleaning, I guess. Again.

That's all we can be together; you're a mechanic and I'm a machine. We won't trust each other fully, and we won't fully avail ourselves of the other's interests and capabilities, but we'll both be safe. We'll both be the same afterward as we were before.

Which is pointless. You need me to help you reframe *your* thinking. We must impress each other.

❖ ❖ ❖

Yes, it sounds ambiguous, but there's a very professional, practical fact to all that warmth and fuzziness: let's both remember that the money that doesn't change hands for full case acceptance when that collaborative bond of trust doesn't happen. I don't make the financial investment if the emotional investment is weak, and not only do you *not* get my case acceptance; chances are, I don't come back to you at all, and worse, it's possible that if my experience is especially negative, other people hear about it through word of mouth or even on the Web:

> The doctors there are caring. They explained to me in detail all my problems and gave me options in my treatment. Everything was totally painless.

> STAY AWAY FROM THIS PLACE, THEY JUST WANT YOUR $$$....unless you want to pay $200 for a cleaning, substandard care, and condescending "dentists." They care more about their profits than their patients. The worst place ever...

Those two reviews appear on a Weblog, one after the other, about the same dentist in my area. No typical note of this kind from patients discusses technique or equipment. (Personally, I'd be eager to post something positive, not so eager to post something negative, because anonymous and brief posts like this are quite unfair. But that doesn't stop anyone from writing them or from reading them and getting an impression.) If we miss our opportunity with each other, and anyone asks about you, I won't tell them about your instruments and your diploma. I'll say, well, we just didn't connect.

Call this frame of thinking anything you like, fuzzy, practical; patient-centered dentistry or unvarnished self-interest. One frame really matters: *Better*. We both want *Better*, capital B. I need to give up my narrow little frame of myself to become *Better*. So do you. I need you to help me imagine my *Better* with me if I can't imagine it alone. I need you to be that ambitious for us both. You want to practice on my mouth? Start on my hopes and fears, on my assumptions, on the needs I barely dare to say aloud.

The guy who sold me my Mercedes understood all of this, believe me.

I'm not asking you to be a car salesman, or a hustler, or to manipulate me into making a dumb decision with ten thousand dollars. I know you're above that as individuals and as a profession. I appreciate that your language and your selling methods are designed to protect us both. But bear in mind that being persuasive, that communicating vividly and with enthusiasm, doesn't make you a hustler. And if we don't understand each other, we aren't just protected from failure and disappointment. We're both protected from real fulfillment. Protected against *Better*—imagine that.

Give me a vision.

Trust yourself, your training, and your high standards to help me make it real.

I don't just need repair. I need renewal, and it can happen in your chair. You need to believe it for me when I don't. Make that spark jump to me.

To do that, you need the best possible vision of yourself. It'll be too much to put in your business card. It won't be on your diploma. I don't know if there's a dental school in the world that can teach you to do that. Like any engineers, you seek to minimize risk, and this is risky. It will change the way you see me, yourself, dentistry, and success.

❖ ❖ ❖

FIVE: GET PAST SELLING

The selling conundrum

You mistrust selling. So do I. Those Mercedes salesmen are ruthless. They home in on your emotional weaknesses, and no matter what's wrong with you, they happen to have the solution right there on the showroom floor. The problem hardly matters. If your parakeet escaped from its cage when you were six, if your date for the prom stood you up, if you're too short for the company basketball team, if your marriage isn't perfect, if the boss doesn't understand you, or if your kids don't listen; let's face it, my friend, your life is a disaster, a catastrophe, and the answer, the salvation, *your last hope*, is a 7-speed automatic transmission with steering-wheel mounted shift paddles, 19 inch aluminum wheels, an Electronic Stability Program, five-passenger seating with generous legroom, and optional Bluetooth connectivity. Happiness comes in seventy-nine custom colors and, of course, white upholstery.

Trust me. Buy this car and your whole life will be better. Sign here. Use my pen.

Believe me, I appreciate any professional who dislikes the idea of selling, because I hate being "sold" for the same reason I can't stand a bad magician. When you can see the extra cards up their sleeves, the tricks are obvious. The lies insult your intelligence. So if you have a deep instinct against selling, thank you.

However, I'd caution you against defining "selling" too broadly. If the shadow of the word obscures some bright ideas you really can use without compromising yourself, then you're not helping either you or me.

It's a conundrum. You need to communicate facts and truths. You need to convey expertise and enthusiasm. And sometimes the line between those things gets blurred. When you step too far to one side or the other, something's wrong, and we both feel it.

❖ ❖ ❖

Going too far

It's better for me and for you that dentistry as a profession errs on the side of caution. The instinct is driven very deep in your professional culture to say too little, because too many dentists in the past said too much. You're still recovering from some of the overstatements and hard-sells that helped give dentistry its negative reputation.

Anyone who wants to understand where all those bad jokes about sadistic shysters in white smocks originated needs only to visit the museum at Temple University's School of Dentistry at Broad Street and Allegheny Avenue in Philadelphia.

One of the exhibits is a bucket filled with thousands of human teeth pulled by a legendary — well, what exactly to call this man is hard to say. To the public, he was the most famous dentist of his time. To the American Dental Association, he was "a menace to the dignity of the profession."

Edgar R.R. "Painless" Parker popularized dentistry by literally turning it into a circus attraction, traveling town-to-town with acrobats and dancing girls. He'd book a theatre, deliver a hellfire-and-brimstone speech on the horrors of bad dental hygiene, and then invite audience members to be treated right there and then as his brass band played. His home office on Flatbush Avenue in New York was pure vaudeville. The street-facing windows were shaded with his portrait. Billboards on the façade declared him to be, "Preeminently par excellent in positively painless perfection practice" and "Particularly pleasing particular patients and philanthropically predisposed to popular prices." How he filled that bucket of teeth is no mystery. He prided himself on speed and volume, touting his record of 357 extractions in one day by wearing them as a necklace. When he was accused of false advertising by calling his practice "painless," he changed his first name legally to Painless!

The dentistry may have been of dubious clinical worth, but the marketing worked terribly well: at his peak, Parker operated 30 dental offices, had 75 dentists on staff, and made $3 million per year.

Today, mercifully, the memory of Dr. Parker is gone, and there isn't a patient on earth who would ask you to readopt his methods. However, in the interest of sterilizing the instruments, so to speak, a couple of Parker's insights have been discarded and discredited when they might bear reevaluation. Parker was a vulgar extremist, a liar, a charlatan and a hazard to the profession and to the patients, certainly. And he was a powerful communicator. He created a dreadful marriage in combining questionable skills with shameless hucksterism, but in cleansing itself of those things, the dental profession may well have thrown out the baby—a vision—with the bathwater.

We have to admit it: Parker had a vision. He wanted patients to have one too. He told them to demand good dentistry as a right, a necessity, something they shouldn't and needn't do without. He shared it so compellingly that people would accept bad dentistry, not knowing the difference. They'd literally let him yank out their teeth on stage with a bugle bleating in their ear. The vision was a lie in practice, of course, and the liar needed to be eradicated, but the vision was true and needed, and it has never been adequately replaced with a finer, more practicable version, even though such a vision can now be upheld truthfully and with integrity by the dental profession every day. If the deep instinct against marketing defines "marketing" so broadly that it dismisses all communication as potential hucksterism, the silence that results is worse than the big talk.

Parker's fault then was in claiming more than he knew. Dentistry's conundrum now is claiming *less* than it knows.

❖ ❖ ❖

A sterile silence

Presumably, every dentist reading this is familiar with Section 5.F. Advertising of the *ADA Principles of Ethics and Code of Professional Conduct:* "Although any dentist may advertise, no dentist shall advertise or solicit patients in any form of communication in a manner that is false or misleading in any material respect."

Before I continue, thanks. Thanks for making this important. Thanks for looking out for me. I know that you and your professional culture have my safety and well-being uppermost in mind with that rule.

That said, however, this rule reminds me of the antibacterial dish detergents you see today on the supermarket shelves. It's hard to argue with a general instinct for cleanliness, but then again, it possible that you're fixing a problem that doesn't really exist, or that the fix is disproportionate, and has itself originated a new problem.

I'd submit to you that the dental profession suffers a kind of Painless Parker hangover. The damage done by such venal practitioners is indisputable and can't ever be tolerated again, but the evolving code of ethics has, before, during and after Parker, promulgated an instinct in responsible dentists for understatement bordering sometimes on paranoia. It's relatively recent that practices of professional advertising have opened up via the ruling in 1977 in *Bates v. State Bar of Arizona* that opened the door to advertising by service providers like you. It's possible that the dental profession, remembering Painless and his ilk, still hasn't embraced the opportunities and challenges of this new openness (and at the same time, it still hasn't fully eradicated the Painless Parkers among you).

Meanwhile, though, many other things have changed for dentists. Your numbers have increased; your training and technology have evolved and improved in orders of magnitude; your place in people's lives is different. But generally, your messaging to people like me is the weak horse running beside these other strong ones. If there's a bone-deep instinct that equates communicating with advertising, and if advertising is presumed to be unethical, then the dentists with the most valuable information may well, as a matter of professionalism, not advertise. From time to time, some go even further, purporting to take an ethical stance on behalf of the patients by going *against* the profession and exposing its flaws. In my reading, I was surprised to find books written under pen names by dentists warning me about the underhanded and unsafe things happening in dental offices. (I don't know quite what to make of them. Would a patient who already fears a dentist read an exposé in search of more reasons to be afraid? Would a willing patient seek to second-guess themselves by reading these books?)

Meanwhile, the near-silence from well-meaning dentists isn't an ethical statement by the dental profession. It's a vacuum, and it just leaves the field open at the extreme for the 21st century Painless Parkers, and to a lesser degree, for those dentists who, with the best intentions, promulgate the mediocre bench ads, flyers and junk mail that seem to be the bulk of today's dentist-patient communication. Any pure, righteous practitioner can be proud for eschewing the low ground, but to say nothing isn't the same as taking the high ground. That dentist might be a genius, an artist and a healer, and she might be right in my neighborhood, but if I don't know she's there, I don't go to her. Meanwhile, I pass half a dozen terrible billboards and bus shelter ads while driving home, and find two cheaply-printed mailers stuffed in my screen door.

Particularly in an era of 24/7 mass communications via every possible device and medium, an instinct for sterile silence has to be questioned. Self-effacing professional scrupulousness has practical limits. If the best dentists in my neighborhood fall silent or if their marketing gets lost in the shuffle among the lesser ones, I'm not served, and neither are the dentists.

❊ ❊ ❊

Let's revisit that ADA rule: "Although any dentist may advertise, no dentist shall advertise or solicit patients in any form of communication in a manner that is false or misleading in any material respect." "Any form of communication" is about as broad a ruling as you can make. At least half your practice is communicating, whether or not you understand that you're doing it—a smile to a patient you happen to see in the local bakery, coaching for the Little League, giving a talk to the Rotary…they all convey impressions about you and about your practice. They all can be very effective solicitations for you, even if you don't intend them that way. On the contrary, if you got arrested for DUI and your name was in the papers, it would very likely affect your reputation in the area. Strictly speaking, of course, that incident has nothing to do with your dental skills, but it falls nevertheless under the broad definition of "any form of communication." It sure communicates to me.

How can you really be responsible for "any form," if I'm the one interpreting what it means?

"False or misleading" is bad, obviously, but sometimes people hear something you haven't actually said, or they hope for something that doesn't materialize. You don't have to outright lie to me if I'm eager to deceive myself. I'm your collaborator, remember, and I need to take responsibility for my role in the success or failure of your practice, just as I ask you to take your responsibility for your role in the success or failure of my healthy mouth. You can't sterilize me against being misled when it's me, not you, doing the misleading.

I'm not addressing that handful of Painless Parker throwbacks out there whose sleazy marketing gives good dentists bad reputations. I am, however, trying to understand what's left to say for the good dentists, the truthful communicators, if they feel so constrained. There's little room to move within the implications of this dictum; if you're good, there's not much latitude to show how and why you're good. Not to mention, of course, that in addition to your freedoms being limited, time is always short. You don't have days at a time to invent clever new marketing concepts. So you fall back on what's conventional, acceptable, tried and adequately proven, even though it might be platitudinous, common and expensive. That would explain why, one day recently, I got flyers from two dentists in my neighborhood. They were originated by the same dental marketing company. They had the same photos, the same text. Only the dentists' names were different. They told me that they were *uniquely* qualified to be my neighborhood dentist—each of them!

I need a dentist, but I didn't call either of them.

Finally, on that ADA rule—the words "in any material respect" are for me to define, as well as for you, and it's entirely likely that what the ADA or a typical dentist considers material, I consider either over my head or immaterial. The dentist friend I mentioned at the beginning of this book felt that the details of his beautiful veneers were thoroughly material, but for me, they were far from the most important thing he needed to say.

If your hands are tied, so are mine. If you and the overseers of the profession, if you and your colleagues, can't come to terms on the hows and whys of communicating, then that distance—the gap—between you and I can't be bridged. You can be accurate and materially truthful within the confines of professional rectitude, and being so can effectively make what you say incomprehensible and immaterial for me. Which is a huge waste for both of us. Your time and money and my benefiting from you are all falling into that gap, and nobody is better off. And with all the possibilities available now to help you communicate honestly and imaginatively, that's simply intolerable.

What *can* you say?

Value propositions are succinct statements that describe what a customer gets from a seller for his money. You read them every day.

Engineers are notorious for conservative, understated value propositions—well, bad ones is what I mean. Their marketing communications tend to be uninspiring, narrow and heavy on the jargon. Engineers are literal, quantitative and factual people by nature, and they're rightly suspicious of anything that taints that mindset— bugs in the computer code or an unproven suggestion. Or emotion, warmth or inspiration. And engineering has almost as much to do with the professional culture of dentistry as medicine does.

As a writer of this kind of communications for companies in telecommunications and software and electrical utilities, I can tell you quite frankly that I have made a pretty decent living writing for engineers, but it's been frustrating for me at times because once I actually understood what they were saying, I realized how much real value my clients had to offer that wasn't being even hinted at. I wanted them to convey some excitement about it. They resisted consistently, believing that the whole value of what they were selling lay in a close, detailed listing of the product specifications. They didn't trust enthusiasm. It doesn't convey the details, and the details are, or seem like, everything there can possibly be to say. I respect that. These people worked hard to learn their skills, and they'd be trivializing their learning and their products and themselves to hide that expertise. The downside, of course, was that they ended up talking mostly to their professional peers, and not necessarily to the people who actually made the buying decisions about the program or the service or the software being offered.

They were the clients, and I was the hired help, so I went along. As a result, there are samples of my work I could show you for which I feel I should be taken out and shot.

"The GCP solution presents a simplified messaging path between the Media Gateway Controllers (MGCs), also referred to as Call Agents (CAs) and Media Gateways (MGs). These device control protocols function in a call control architecture consisting of signaling gateways, which are responsible for PSTN control and intelligent MGCs, controlling reduced intelligence MGs."

Yes, I wrote that. Please hold your applause.

❖ ❖ ❖

The term "value proposition" is relatively new, but the idea is as old as what you do. All the Hippocratic Oath is, is a value proposition. It talks about you in your business relationship with me, implying in each word and between every line that I, the patient, am real (if that sounds obvious, take my word, many patients do not feel real to their health care providers, and many providers don't care); that I have challenges before me that you can remediate; that you have to hold yourself to high standards of conduct to do it; and that should you fail to keep those standards, you break the bond between us that you aspire to uphold, and therefore break the oath.

You revere the words of the oath for their long history and for their sanctity in your vocation. From my angle, Hippocrates was a business writer. A great one, in fact. Two thousand three hundred years after the initial version, after numerous translations and alterations, and the business practicality of that oath is still as hard and bright as a steel probe.

Everything else has changed in those twenty-three centuries, but the *character* of the practitioner is still front-and-center. The Oath doesn't just tell you just to *have* that character. It tells you to *use* it. Humble as Hippocratic medicine is, permitting nature to lead in the healing process, you must apply what you have— "all measures [that] are required, avoiding those twin traps of overtreatment and therapeutic nihilism" as Dr. Lasagna put it. Those aren't the only traps, as we've seen. Overmarketing or undermarketing, unexamined assumptions about what is and what isn't of value to a patient, or simple inattention; the traps are all over your practice. You don't need to be a nihilist to violate the Oath. You just need to give up asking how to communicate your value, to settle into easy habits, lower your standards a little, and give up having fun. Treat your patients as the "filling at four." You might even get away with it if your patients assume that all dentists are like that.

Of course, that's only until they hear about one in your neighborhood who isn't.

Hippocrates and his successors keep challenging you not just to deliver service of the highest caliber, but to invest everything of yourself that's worth it for me, the patient, to see. It's all there in that uncompromising, elegant writing.

I will remember that there is art to medicine as well as science, and that warmth, sympathy, and understanding may outweigh the surgeon's knife or the chemist's drug.

I will not be ashamed to say "I know not," nor will I fail to call in my colleagues when the skills of another are needed for a patient's recovery.

I will prevent disease whenever I can, for prevention is preferable to cure.

Roughly translated, "warmth" in Latin is *aestuo.* "Sympathy" is *sympathīa.* Understanding is *astutia.* They aren't on your diploma. I know you have excellent equipment, but these tools are more effective competitive advantages, and they're yours free, if you'll take them. If you use them for me, they will outweigh the surgeon's knife or the chemist's drug. If you use them for yourself, they will outweigh any need for generic messages a marketing agency gives you, not to mention the need to pay what they charge you for their services.

❖ ❖ ❖

Your GUI: how to say what you can say

Ironically, one of the most important and elegant solutions to the kind of gap we're discussing here happened in one of the most ruthlessly technical of all industries. Everyone reading this uses this solution all the time: the graphical user interface, known by its acronym, the GUI.

Those of you old enough to remember the first personal computers remember the screen that opened with a C-prompt and a blinking cursor: C:\>_. You had to understand MS-DOS, the old operating system for personal computers, or else you couldn't tell the computer what you wanted it to do.

Those who took the trouble to learn fell in love with computers, but for the rest of us, we quite didn't get the point. These machines were both highly capable and utterly obtuse. If you typed in the instruction incorrectly, even by just one character, the thing just sat there blinking at you with that infuriating C:\>_, C:\>_, C:\>_. It was reason enough for lots of people to just ignore computers, and for those of us who tried and failed with them, to conduct experiments involving gravity, five-story buildings, and the IBM Aptiva.

Apple and then Microsoft changed all that by creating the GUI. They didn't abandon the underlying code; they just put a friendly face over it. They gave us little icons that any user could understand: a trash can for things you wanted to throw away, color-coded symbols for the program you wanted to start. It was simple. It was friendly. Anyone could understand it, and because anyone could, immediately anyone did, unlocking for themselves all that power and productivity that had been sitting unused. That was only about thirty years ago, and you know what happened: the greatest revolution in the workplace since the electric light. Apple and Microsoft changed themselves and thereby changed the rest of us.

I know I don't have to tell you what happened to the value of the companies.

They didn't compromise any of the machine's functionality by creating the GUI. They didn't water anything down, didn't cheapen anything. They recognized that value of the machine was compromised by its value proposition, which with the old DOS screens, was simple: I'm a computer. You work for me, on my terms. If you don't know my terms, go away.

Much as the communications from engineers do. And like the one by dentists who, with the best intentions, want to tell you the details about porcelain veneers.

The GUI flipped that around. Now the computer asked, "How can I help?" Or as one of Microsoft's ad slogans said, "Where do you want to go today?" This obnoxious little box that used to turn up its nose at you had become an eager friend, a magic carpet, your obedient genie.

Anyone who dismisses the practicality of friendliness should remind themselves that a share of Microsoft bought in 1985 has split nine times. I hear that Gates kid did pretty well too.

"Where do you want to go today?" What a daring expression of commitment—and it's utterly different from a typical engineer's statement of value. It's open ended, vague, imprecise and ambiguous. It doesn't set terms, it asks you for *your* terms. It tells you that *you* decide what this machine is, what it does, what it's worth. You control it, not vice versa. It's flexible and adaptable and it makes you more capable as you want. We made this product, and we know it far better than you ever will. But you bought this product. Who decides its value?

You do.

❖ ❖ ❖

Do you know what your value is to your patients?

Do you have a GUI mindset that reaches out on the user's terms, or do you ask them to understand you so they can use you?

I appreciate that your training has always been subject to peer review and rigorous supervision, and I'm grateful that the profession polices itself to keep the Painless Parkers out, or at least suppressed. But this is personal, far less scientific than dentist-to-dentist discourse, and there's a line you feel intuitively you can approach but not cross. Talk too much about your practice, your skills, your office, your instrumentation, and you lose me. Hard sell on price and you seem unprofessional. Perhaps worse than these, let someone else do your talking for you, and spend a lot of money with results that make you look completely generic, and have your flyer arrive in my mailbox the same day as this week's specials at my supermarket, *Newsweek*, two bills, and a flyer from another dentist.

Try doing this without preconceptions: think about the role you've played, and want to play, in your patient's lives. Think about it from their point of view, not yours or your peers'. Take some notes. Toss out your first words if they sound too much like something you heard in school or in a professional seminar. Ask your spouse or a friend for feedback. Think like a customer, not like a seller, and remember how you react when someone is bearing down too hard on you to buy something, and when you're delighted beyond your expectations. I'm asking you to take time for this. You won't just be putting down a few ideas you can use in communicating with patients (chances are a marketing firm you hire, if you have one, will resist your ideas, or just misunderstand what you do; after all, they're the experts at marketing—but how many of them really understand dentistry? And if the dentist with no experience and an engineering mindset is directing their efforts, then the blind are leading the blind). You might be asking yourself questions you haven't thought of for some time, and reconnecting with the best reasons why you became a dentist at all.

Use the Oath as a starting point. I can't imagine a better way to reconcile your commitment to my well-being with the health of your business.

And please, don't treat this as some sort of fluffy exercise. You're looking for case acceptance, right? If you don't understand my *entire* case, how will you get me to accept the entirety of what you have in mind for me?

So tell me, what is your value proposition? What's mine? What's ours?

❖ ❖ ❖

SIX: THE PARTS AND THE WHOLE OF OUR PRACTICE

The parts of me

I'm a single name in your appointment book, but I'm six or seven different people in your waiting room. This is especially so if I'm a new patient who doesn't know you. How you deal with that makes all the difference for our relationship.

With some dentists, the "me" you see never changes, because our relationship never gets past the superficial—"Good morning, open please"—that's about it. I suspect there are dentists who like it this way. They don't want to be my psychologist or my facilitator or whatever else I might hope for. Fair enough. I don't want to be their financial benefactor. They'll never treat me for anything above the absolute minimum.

Those dentists who seek to know more about me have a much better chance at achieving case acceptance from me. Frankly, while I hope they might be doing it either out of deep human compassion, I know it's more likely coming from sheer business practicality, i.e., greed. No problem–either one works for me, if the results are there. And really, I believe that even if the human compassion isn't there at the outset, it will be soon enough. It works like a smile works. Start today as a greedy cynic, if that's who you are. But if you've ever been gratified by the work you do, you want it again, and the more it comes to you, the more you grow as a person from it. You can't stay cynical if the satisfaction you get helps you grow. That your practice grows as well confirms the point. The dentists who want quick paybacks from their patients are like the day traders making a million one day and losing it the next. They constantly need to waste time and money replacing the patients who walk away. The astute investors understand my growth, their growth and business growth, and they know how to make all those happen.

So I'm in your waiting room. One person, ten or so different parts. I can hold about that many contradictory ideas in mind, and all of them will affect your capacity to treat me to the level you'd like. Some dentists treat one, two maybe. Some address them all because they look for them.

I fall into a couple of categories. Allow me to introduce myselves.

Part of me absolutely does not want to be here. I don't care about the pain that made me call you. I'd medicate myself with horse liniment right now, if I could. My blood pressure is up, my heart's thudding. I have goose bumps. I'm fighting with myself just to stay here.

Part of me fully appreciates that seeking your care is the sensible, adult thing to do.

Part of me hears that high-pitched whine coming from the drilling underway in the other room, and that part would rather you just decapitate me and get it over with.

Let's say the situation is less urgent. A friend recommended that I ask you about cosmetic work, so I'm here for a consultation. Part of me hears my friend telling me how nice I'd look with a little help from you, and that I might be happier, and meet someone special and feel great. And part of me knows I don't really deserve that kind of happiness, that it's rare and precious and you can't just go purchase it, and that I might as well find a substitute for it. With 19 inch aluminum wheels. I'll let a version of happiness get as close as my driveway, but making it part of me, well…that's too much to hope for.

In the first case, the tradeoff is fairly simple. I'll endure some additional pain and suffering, reluctantly, if you can remove the pain and suffering I brought with me. The second case is more complicated. *I'll actually resist you if you try to do me good.* The perfectly logical part of you is talking calmly with the perfectly logical part of me, but I'm about 10% perfectly logical. That's the part you see nodding thoughtfully while you're talking about the procedures you'd like me to accept. The other 90% is thinking of any possible excuse to say no. While the logical 10% sits with you, the other 90% is outside your office in an underground bunker surrounded by sandbags and antiaircraft guns. I'm telling myself that only beautiful people ever get a smile like the one you're showing me. I'm picturing syringes the size of whaling harpoons. I'm calculating the absolutely impossible finances of what you're proposing, and I'm seeing my 19 inch wheels of happiness sitting in *your* driveway.

Am I wrong about all this? Of course. Does that keep me from walking out of your office and never coming back? Of course not. The majority rules, right or wrong. I'm taking a vote here, and the 90% of me that's wrong or misguided or ill-informed or afraid wins, regardless of how bad the decision happens to be.

Welcome to me. Obviously, I'm in conflict with myself. Oddly enough, though, all the parts of me want the same things. We just need to be reminded. The part that fears you and wants to leave your office wants my safety, health and well-being. So does the part that keeps me there waiting for you. The part that squanders money on a hot new car wants self-esteem. So does the part that envies those beautiful people in all your photos of smiling faces. Getting all these various parts to a common understanding is possible, but if you don't address all of me, which is to say all of us, none of us will end up paying for you.

❖ ❖ ❖

The parts of you

By "you," I mean all of you. If you're asking me to give you permission to make changes to all of me, then you need to be all of you. The dentist is part of you. The person you are is the rest. Bring them all.

What else are you, besides being a dentist? Who else are you?

Your training, I would hope, ought to have enhanced the other best aspects of you, and helped you set aside those parts of you that are incompatible with performing at the level you at which you want to work. Be careful, though, in making that evaluation of what matters and what doesn't. Something that you feel is superficial or unnecessary to excellent dentistry might be exactly what I need to see. (I'll say it again—excellent dentistry happens only when we to work together. Neither of us does it on our own.)

Call it empathy, but it's more complicated than that, and more selfish too, and the selfishness is a good thing. Not selfishness precisely, but self-interest for sure. Your comprehensive understanding of me is a practical clinical and business tool that helps us both. If you've ever been an impatient customer, for example, I can use that. If you've ever felt frustrated by jargon (possibly it was something I wrote) or by unclear directions from an expert, I can use that. Somewhere in your experiences are feelings just like the ones that conflict within me as I sit in your waiting room. You have the same debates going on within yourself that I have in me. You've been a patient, a customer, a suitor, a doubter, a hopeful human being reaching for a miracle just as I'm reaching for one, and you remember what it's like to feel both fear and desire at once. You have money to spend and choices to make. You have crazy priorities sometimes, and sometimes common sense rules.

We have these things in common.

They're your GUI. They're what will make a good impression on me. They're the bridge between us. And if you leave them at home when you go to work, you're neglecting instruments that could work for you as effectively as anything on the tray beside your chair. These similarities might all be open lanes on a wide bridge between us as we try to understand each other, and even the seemingly irrelevant ones are valuable. Narrow yourself down to just one lane, your expertise as a dentist, and you might close off all these other opportunities for us to share, learn, and invest ourselves together. Use them and, well, it's simple. I understand you because you understand me.

Now you're "my" dentist. Now we can share a vision.

All your parts have value

You're a dentist, a teacher and a student. And under that white smock, you're a son or a daughter, and maybe a parent and a sibling. You're a customer and a vendor of services. You're an entrepreneur, an employer and an investor. You speak and you listen. The roles you play in a typical week inside and outside the office overlap hugely with the ones I play. And like me, you hear your own internal parts yapping in conflict: the craftsman who wants to sculpt a work of dental art and the businessperson who has to keep an eye on throughput and the day's appointments; the novice who is being thrilled and excited by dentistry, and, sadly, the mid-career practitioner who feels stuck and bored by it. Nothing is irrelevant *per se*; there will be a moment during our interaction where the part of you that really reaches me is the understanding sibling or the good neighbor. It might be that moment, not the quality of your porcelain veneers, that tips my decision to commit to an expensive course of care.

Yes, it's counterintuitive. You spent years becoming an expert, but there are instances in our collaboration when your expertise may actually work against you, and thus against me, if you let it. There are moments when it does more to separate us than it does to bring us together. If it's intimidating instead of informative, if you seem to understand just one part of me as an expert and nothing else of me as a human being, we're further apart, not closer.

What is the likelihood of our mutual success if the fearful part of me is met by the part of you that's impatient that day, or the part that speaks in jargon, or the one that's bored and wants to be golfing? Our affinity is blocked if the wrong parts meet. If I feel confused, neglected, marginalized, trivialized or just not really seen—if I'm just the "filling at four"—you couldn't sell me water if I were dying of thirst. If the understanding we both need is there, I'm listening. I'm granting trust. I'm investing. I can walk out of your office throbbing, drooling and numb down to the waist, and if I'm thinking *I'm glad I came,* I'll be back. On the other hand, I can walk out pain-free with a perfect technical outcome, and if for any reason I'm thinking *I wish I hadn't come*—we just didn't connect—you've seen me for the last time. My feeling might have nothing at all to do with the procedure. That I was understood, and that I was invited to understand *you*, matters more. That I see this as part of a process toward a better goal is part of what gets me to accept that goal.

It's this simple: if you want case acceptance, make your case. Making it to the professor you had in dental school or to your peers and colleagues won't do. You need to make it to *me*, and keep in mind, I may well be in complete disagreement with myself when you begin.

❖ ❖ ❖

Rapport

We're talking about *rapport* here. Forgive me for giving the definition, but it's important to what we're sharing: "relationship, especially one of mutual trust or emotional affinity." Dr. Lasagna thought it was significant enough to mention it in his poetic version of your Hippocratic Oath: "warmth, sympathy, and understanding." A really effective dentist can put that on his or her business card. The bad ones can't find it with a map even if they graduated *summa cum laude* from dental school.

The ancient Greeks called their healing centers *asklepions* after Asclepius, the god of healing. Particular attention was paid at these places to the ambiance and beauty of the setting. Even three thousand years ago, they understood the value of getting the patient to relax. The patient would spend time just getting acclimated, attending plays to lift his spirits, and setting worry aside. Then he would consult with a priest. Speaking scientifically, it went downhill from here. The therapies involved potions and snakes.

Luckily for those who followed, Hippocratic medicine was being practiced along with this cultist school, and healing techniques based on empiricism and the observation of nature eventually won out, more or less. But the witch doctors understood what Painless Parker knew much later on. A little theatre is a good thing, if it helps to motivate and comfort the patient. Let's remember also the billions of dollars spent every year by modern Americans on "alternative" treatments because they fear or mistrust the mainstream, and that some of these treatments would be improved by the presence of a shaman and a snake. Dentistry as a profession has worked hard to elevate itself out of the era when a dental degree sold for $20. Sadly, plenty of people holding dime-store credentials still ply their trades for a gullible public. The reason why people buy them is obvious: the sellers indulge the buyers' craving for warmth, empathy and understanding. Big medicine has become disengaged medicine. It's cold.

❖ ❖ ❖

You can't order good impressions out of a catalog. How do you make them?

Start with a typical appointment. It might be the first, the fifth, the twentieth, you name it. I'm already negotiating with myself about what I'll accept from you. There's an order in my mind.

At the top of my priorities is my safety. When I'm in your office, I'm on high alert from pure survival instinct, and believe me, if you could perform whatever it is you're about to do for me by waving a wand and not touching me at all, I'd ask for that. You know I value safety. What are you doing to address that? The white smock, the appearances of professionalism of your people, the cleanliness and order of the office are all good and all basic. If you're friendly and calm, if you take a moment to show me what you need to do and why it matters, if you give me good information about what to expect, I can feel those concerns subside. The other sides emerge: *I'm worried about my safety* recedes and *I'm in good hands* comes up. *I don't understand what's happening* backs off and *I know this is for the best* arises.

Good effects. I know them when they're really there.

My values aren't changing here. What's happening is that you're addressing them on my terms. And you're reconciling them with your own values.

Let me see that.

❖ ❖ ❖

Five minutes for rapport

The five minutes you spend managing your one-to-one relationship with me helps both you and me to reach the goals of that immediate appointment, even if it's just a cleaning. It's also a very practical demonstration of the mutuality of our goals, and a reason for me to call you my dentist. I'll listen to your proposals for more elaborate courses of care when we're in that state.

Simple question: how much eye contact do we make during a typical appointment?

I asked myself this last time I saw my former dentist. I knew I was being a little unfair to him, because we never really had much of a relationship during the two years I was his patient. For me to expect him to greet me like some old friend would have been silly.

His assistant once tried persuading me to ask him about veneers—"he's the veneer guy," she told me. He might be; I never asked him. But I'm getting ahead of myself here. Eye contact—the answer is, we didn't have any. Typically, he was in the back when I came into the office. I sat in the waiting room. His assistant conducted me to the chair. She put the bib on me, laid out the instruments, set up my chart and x-rays, and left me alone to wait. I brought something to read with me, because sitting there for ten minutes or so, sometimes longer, gave me the chance I so badly wanted to catch up on the coverage of Britney Spears' marriage in a six-month old *People* magazine. I listened to ringing phones and heard footsteps behind me and wondered if they'd forgotten I was there.

You might try sitting in your chair sometime and contemplating a neat array of shiny picks, hooks, spatulas, carvers, scrapers and mirrors a foot away. Lay a hypo beside them to get the full effect. You'll actually *want* to read about Britney Spears.

Anyway, after a few minutes of *People*, the dentist would come, sit beside me, and start working. There might be a couple of perfunctory words exchanged, but generally the interaction was efficient and focused. The strict goals of the appointment were fulfilled; if I was there for a cleaning, I got a cleaning. If I was there for a filling, I got a filling.

The lamp over my former dentist's chair is a MedCon GProma by Daray Lighting, Ltd. I had plenty of time to memorize that information before and during the time the dentist was working. Our time spent talking was as close to zero as he could make it, and obviously there wasn't any dialogue while he was working, so the little details of his office registered, but I couldn't tell you today what color his eyes are, and I know he wouldn't recognize me if we passed on the street.

Simple question again: how much eye contact do we make during a typical appointment? Why do I ask?

Because that's rapport time, meaning teaching time, encouragement time, persuasion time and yes, selling time. That's when you share your vision. Eye-to-eye, that's when you're *my* dentist.

That five minutes never happened between me and my former dentist. Neither did any case acceptance.

You could diagram a typical experience, and see whether it's there and how much there is during an appointment:

Eye Contact	Minutes
Patient to receptionist	5
Patient to *People*	10
Patient to assistant	6
Patient in chair alone with Britney	10*
Patient to MedCon GProma dental operating light by Daray Lighting, Ltd., while dentist works	30-60
Patient to dentist	1
Patient to MasterCard bill	1

*feels like three days

I'm being flippant here, I know. Sorry. But this chart isn't far off the truth, and this question is very serious: when are you making your money? I can tell you when you *aren't* making it: when I'm reading *People* or memorizing logos on your instruments, you aren't.

No kidding—walk through your office some time from place to place and look at what I see during my typical appointment. When you're facing me, listening to me, inquiring about me, counseling and encouraging me, you are. It wouldn't take a huge shift in the time spent to make that change, just a few minutes, but given every other painful experience that occurs during this hour, with *People* at the top of the pain list, might it not be good for us both if I left your office feeling that I'm important to you, that we understand each other, and intrigued and optimistic about your ongoing treatment plan instead of just numb?

Is that worth doing for you? It would be for me, and if you'll permit a patient to say so, it would be good for our practice, too.

❖ ❖ ❖

SEVEN: SHARING YOUR BEST TO CREATE MINE

You must come home some evenings feeling great about what you did that day. What makes you feel like that?

I'd bet it wasn't the actual treatment you provided, though that was obviously part of it. Presumably, it was seeing the good effects we've been talking about. Your version of Ms. Johnson stopped by to tell you something wonderful that happened because of the change you made for her, and you felt affirmed in every fond hope you had for your practice.

I hope that happens a lot. What do you do with a story like that? With whom do you share it? How do you tell it? How does it help me, your prospective patient, and you, the entrepreneur?

That conversation I mentioned before, the one between the dentist and the patient away from the chair—that's one setting where you can use it. I'd ask you, though, to think about what you want the outcome of that conversation to be. The few minutes this interaction takes could make all the difference in my acceptance of your treatment plan, so invest some time now, before we talk. I don't mean you should rehearse responses to questions I might have. Any patient knows a canned answer when a dentist gives one, and for me, that's a deal-breaker. Someone who gives a mechanical answer to a simple question must be a mechanic. Even real mechanics don't do that. Just ask yourself how you feel about what I'm asking, and if you would, answer some questions that will help us both.

- When did you first want to be a dentist? What gave you that idea? What did it feel like to decide?
- Who among your instructors did you find inspiring? What about this person was interesting to you? What would you say was the most important thing you learned from this instructor— was it a personal lesson or a professional one, or both?

- Was there a classmate or a colleague whom you found particularly noteworthy? Why? Was there someone from this time whose enthusiasm you admired?

- Think about a few great experiences you've had as a student and as a practitioner. What about them made them memorable for you? How did they improve the lives of the patients you treated? What differences did you make for them? How did that make you feel?

- Do you still get that feeling of pride and satisfaction? What gives it to you? When did it last happen, and why?

- Athletes and artists talk about a "zone" when they feel an indescribable kind of oneness with the situation they're in or the work they're doing, and everything clicked. Have you ever experienced that, inside or outside your office?

- What would you hope to hear your patients say about you? What can you do today to make that happen?

- How is being a dentist helping you fulfill your life goals? Is it helping you grow personally? Is it helping you meet your financial expectations? Is it helpful to you in your personal relationships? Has it been a cause for your growth as a person, even spiritually? Can you see that happening? How?

- What excites you about it? If I asked you to tell me some things you truly love about being a dentist, about dentistry, even about the technology and tools of it, what would you say?

- What stories can you (or the team in your office) tell me about your best cases, your most satisfying successes? What gives you that feeling of deepest satisfaction?

- Is it clear to anyone who comes to you that your team members like and trust you? How is that conveyed?

If you shared all this with me, I'd listen carefully to your answers with genuine respect, but this is just like the conversation I had with my dentist friend before—the fact and the details aren't important to me, to be frank, but your passion, enthusiasm, and delight speak volumes. I want to know very much that you're in touch with the best feelings you have about yourself, your career, your practice and your results. I need to see that light in your eyes when we talk. I need to see your face glow a little and to understand that you really do like what you do, that you aren't one of the ones who'd rather be golfing or doing something else entirely. I need to know that my dentist loves what he or she does. There might well be a better technician in the same medical building you're in, but if that dentist is just a dispassionate technician, and I'm looking to invest some serious time and money, you win. You care more. You enjoy more. You relish what you do and that means everything to me.

How much should you tell me about yourself? Next to nothing. I know it sounds like I'm contradicting myself, but I'm not. You can communicate volumes to me without saying much at all directly about you. You do it by asking about me, by listening actively, by encouraging me, by telling me explicitly and implicitly that you understand my apprehensions, my doubts, and that I have a dream or a hope I left behind.

This might make you uncomfortable. Maybe you'd feel you aren't really talking about dentistry. I disagree — to me that's exactly what you're talking about. Look at it this way...

When you confine yourself to the facts and details of your work, you're inside your comfort zone. It feels right to speak in these terms because it's precise, and accurate, and factual, and all those traits have always been part of your training, right? Whether it was in dental school or on some form of continuing education, the facts and the details were the bull's-eye, so to speak. Like this one. If you were hitting that, you were doing the right thing. Other issues like these patient hopes and aspirations I'm talking about are all peripheral.

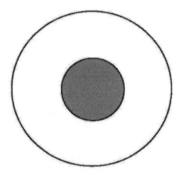

Those are the effects. You can't predict them. You can't even aim at them. From my point of view, though, that target is reversed, like this:

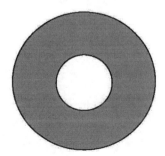

The periphery *is* the bull's eye. The center is the details of dentistry. And that's not why I'm there. The center is process, technology, materials, and the MedCon GProma by Daray Lighting. They are at best considerations for the process, and frankly I want to take as little interest in the process as I can. But the periphery is my life, my whole messy life. The little space in the middle is where you do your work. That humongous, scary gray area outside that is where you have your effects.

That is dentistry.

Here's your real work address. It isn't the one on your business card.

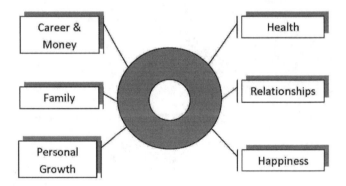

Under each of those headings are issues you address, indirectly but with truth and power. My teeth are the tip of my personal iceberg. When you change them, you change what lies below the surface, in my bull's eyes:

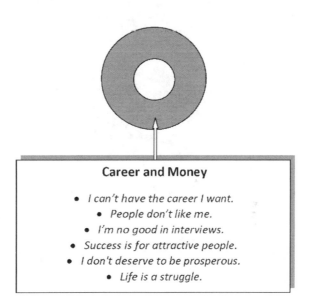

Career and Money

- *I can't have the career I want.*
  - *People don't like me.*
- *I'm no good in interviews.*
- *Success is for attractive people.*
- *I don't deserve to be prosperous.*
  - *Life is a struggle.*

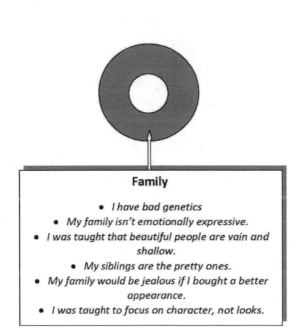

Family

- *I have bad genetics*
- *My family isn't emotionally expressive.*
- *I was taught that beautiful people are vain and shallow.*
- *My siblings are the pretty ones.*
- *My family would be jealous if I bought a better appearance.*
- *I was taught to focus on character, not looks.*

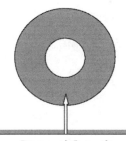

Personal Growth

- *I'm afraid to be seen as I am.*
- *I am not worthy of success.*
- *People like me are supposed to be lonely.*
- *I never get what I want.*
- *I'm not up to life's challenges.*
- *I'm stuck with the life I have.*

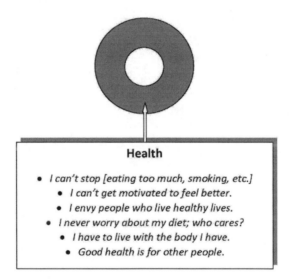

Health

- *I can't stop [eating too much, smoking, etc.]*
  - *I can't get motivated to feel better.*
  - *I envy people who live healthy lives.*
- *I never worry about my diet; who cares?*
  - *I have to live with the body I have.*
  - *Good health is for other people.*

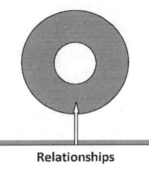

Relationships

- *Love is for beautiful people—not for me.*
- *Nobody wants me the way I am, and I can't change that.*
- *I'm going to die alone.*
- *My last lover left me for someone more attractive.*
- *I gave up trying to be good-looking.*
- *I'm intimidated by people more attractive than I am, so I don't get close to anyone.*

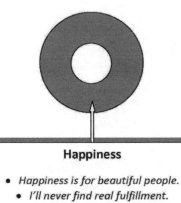

Happiness

- *Happiness is for beautiful people.*
- *I'll never find real fulfillment.*
- *I fear feeling too good because it doesn't last.*
- *You can't make a smile that I really believe in.*
- *I wasn't meant to be happy.*
- *Real happiness is for someone else.*

Those doubts, fears, and terrible decisions, all those *I can'ts* and *I'll nevers,* all those sad, sorry, unnecessary surrenders I made, and all the very real effects those all have on my physical health—those are what you're treating when you build me a new smile.

How do you communicate to me that you understand issues like these? Easy: leave the facts aside and tell me the truth. Tell me anecdotes, not about the techniques and materials you use, but about the effects you've had on people. You don't need to brag about it; you don't need to go into the tiny details or compromise any confidentiality, but somewhere in your experience is a Ms. Johnson whose case resembles mine.

Somewhere in there is an instance where the work you did made a difference in someone's career, where you helped someone find that spark of motivation that started a diet or a relationship.

Someone among your patients got married because of what you did.

Someone lost forty pounds.

Someone quit smoking.

There's a patient whose family life you changed.

There's one whose health you transformed.

There might be someone whose life you saved.

If personal growth and happiness sound outside your scope, think again, because I'd bet there's a smile of yours walking around that made the bearer feel like the sun had come up in their lives for the first time in a long time.

Where and how to share

I just asked you to take five minutes in your office to talk with me, and here I am asking you to tell me detailed stories that would take much longer to share. It's extra work, I know, but for the sake of our practice, I'd ask you to evaluate some additional possibilities you can use to communicate with me.

If it seems a little daunting, look at it this way: most of your competition won't even try this. Most of the work required happens at the beginning of the process. As you learn, it gets less expensive in time and money to do it, and it has one great advantage over anything you could buy from an agency or a flyer company: it's yours.

- **Print**: If you pay for professional marketing, it's worth considering just how well it reflects who you really are. The samples I collected in my research indicate that marketing firms assemble newsletters out of generic short pieces, and then personalize them with the client dentist's name and address. Generic is just that, generic. I know I should floss, thanks. I *don't* know that you understand your true value for me, though. So I'd rather get something that looks a little amateurish if it tells me more about who you are, what you know about the effects you have, and how you can make my life better. You can buy inexpensive newsletter software for under $100 and set up simple templates that, once completed, make it easy for you to send out mass mailings to your client list. Have you added new technology to your office? Do your patients know your staff? Did you read something in the journals or even in the news that might be of use to your patients? Is there a story you can share about some case you know of (of course without revealing patient information)?

An additional advantage of this kind of newsletter is that you don't need to print it at all. You can send it in Portable Document Format, or .pdf, as an attachment to a bulk email. No postage, no printing costs, unless you decide to have some made up for your waiting room.

Three or four times a year is about right. More than that and it's too much work for us both.

- **Web**: Web sites are very practical for certain transactions, but there are a couple of downsides I can think of as they relate to your practice. They aren't necessarily local, so you're competing for attention with dentists from all over the world. But then again, if you're developing content like articles or short advice items for the newsletter, they'll work here too.

- **Podcasts**: Podcasting is a relatively new as a marketing medium, involving brief digital audio files. It'll take an investment of a little time for you to get acquainted with the equipment needs and distribution channels, but if you have a good voice, and some good stories and advice to share, you might be among the first dentists to try it. The audio files can help provide content for a Web site too.

- **Speaking engagements**: Even if you live in a small town, you have Rotary, Elks, Toastmasters chapters, gyms and fitness centers, church groups, and companies around you. Everything we've been discussing here could make a very credible and informative lunch-and-learn or after-work session for them, if you ask for a chance to talk with them. Obviously you have in mind to meet people in the community and to build your practice, but that's not how you want to make this offer. From their point of view, a health care professional visiting to discuss good overall well-being, habit control over smoking or drinking, diet and exercise, is a win for them, because bad employee habits are bad news for a company's health care costs and absenteeism, and for a health club's members. Let them know that you're there to talk about *them*, not about you and your practice, and go with a prepared talk, even with a PowerPoint or some easy-to-make presentation, and talk about preventive care of the mouth as the best way to take care of the whole body. Keep it about *them*—if you talk about dentistry, remember, talk about effects.

The "don'ts" of these media are simple to list:

- Don't scold people about bad dental habits. They aren't listening to you so they'll feel worse.

- Own the effects of your work but make the patient the hero.

- Don't show clinical photos of before-and-afters—show only results photos, and make sure to show the patient's eyes. The mouth may be where you work, but the eyes—that's where I'll understand the real effects of what you did.

- Make sure as well that if you use patient photos, you have that patient's written permission.
- Above all, don't hard sell.

The "dos" are easy too: be a friend. Seek their trust. Show them that you have a vision for them. Smile. Look them in the eye, even in your writing—write in the second person about "you," just as I'm doing here. Anticipate the questions you want to hear and be ready to engage them sincerely with real answers, not canned ones. Remember your passion. Communicate your caring and commitment over your expertise.

The disadvantages to all these media are that you need to invest time, particularly in starting up, but that diminishes as you become more proficient. The real challenge is that you're doing something few dentists do: you're speaking for yourself.

❖ ❖ ❖

The order of the story

One more idea to keep in mind: you're used to working and planning in linear fashion, A→B→C. You make a diagnosis, lay out a treatment plan, and possibly suggest a result. Some of you have imaging equipment to help a patient visualize the way they'll look when you're through.

The path between the past and the future—stage B—isn't what matters to me. B is the realm of the immediate: diagnosis, assessment, interpretation and treatment design. This is much too confining for what I need our relationship to be. This is a mechanic's conversation, frankly. Most of the conversations I've ever had with a dentist were like this. They were brief, technical, and impersonal. I barely understood them, and if I cared about the message, it was because I expected pain and financial expense to be part of it. What I wanted to get my arms around was C. C is the end result, and I need to believe as deeply and as quickly as I can that that beautiful future me is true *right now*.

Our conversation should go A→C→B, past→ future→present. I live in A, or more precisely, I live *with* A and prolong it. My whole past is written in my mouth, in the smile I hide, in the fears I feel to show it. I want to leave that behind as quickly as I can.

Your opportunity is to help me do that. Take me to the future. Tell me about someone like me who you changed, and I'm seeing myself changed that way. I'm feeling new possibilities for my life. If those possibilities are real, we can discuss B, the details of how we'll do that in collaboration. Make the possibilities irresistibly real and I'll say yes.

Here are a few examples, based on hypothetical cases.

Work and Career

A patient I know is a public prosecutor in the local office of the District Attorney, and she mentioned to me that she was having trouble talking with juries during her trials.

If you've ever served on a jury, you understand that the attorneys try to establish a friendly relationship with the people sitting in judgment of the case. If the attorneys fail at that, or worse, if they give you the impression that they're untrustworthy, then they're less likely to win the case.

I noticed that she held her hand up in front of her mouth as she talked. She felt embarrassed by her smile. Here she was, a smart, accomplished lawyer, and her reservations about her appearance were getting in the way.

It takes just a couple of office visits for someone to improve their smile, and so she started seeing the results fairly quickly in her work. She told me she felt new confidence in talking to her juries. With her new smile, she's more comfortable standing close to them, looking them face-to-face and building that rapport she needs to make her arguments.

Family

I ran into the son of one of my patients at church, and he told me, "Thanks for giving us our father back."

I asked him what he meant, and he explained, "He used to be active and outgoing, but in the last few years when he was having problems with his mouth he just wasn't the same man. You just gave him a set of restorations, and it took ten years off his face. He's like a new man, or really, he's like the guy he was—he's out with Mom and the grandkids, he's socializing with the neighbors, and he's walking two miles every night and losing weight. We were really concerned that he was wasting away; we were worried he was clinically depressed and had just given up on life. You gave him back to us." That's the kind of story that makes me grateful to be a dentist.

Personal Growth

One of my new patients just shared this with me: "The company I've worked for my whole career," he said, "has a requirement that senior executives travel to our regional offices giving speeches and updates to our field staff. I've passed up on promotions twice, even refusing raises and bonuses. When my third opportunity came up, they gave me an ultimatum: take the promotion or find another job.

"I didn't want the promotions because I dreaded speaking in public. What made me afraid to talk with large groups? Simple—I hated how I looked. I've always been self-conscious about my teeth, but in my family we were raised to think it was just vanity to spend a lot of money on your looks. Finally, though, with a couple of kids heading for college, I couldn't refuse more income, and I came to you.

"I wish I'd done this twenty years ago. I'm not just a better executive now—I'm a better person. I feel eager to share what I know with our younger employees and I relish the chances I get to talk with them one-to-one, or three hundred of them at a time. I can be a mentor now. I can be a leader for them. I had no idea how much of a difference this could make for me."

Health

This doesn't happen often, thank God, but when it does, I feel like I've made a real difference.

A patient of mine is a young man in great shape—a marathon runner, a long-distance bicyclist, in the prime of his life. He doesn't smoke, doesn't drink; I mean, there's no reason for a guy like this to worry about his health. He goes in for a standard annual physical and in half an hour, he comes out with a clean bill.

Well, he was in for a cleaning with me and I saw some small leukoplakia. I told him what they are and what they might mean. We called his doctor immediately and he went back for tests. Yes, it was cancer, but because we caught it so early, his outlook is very good. His doctor called me back to give me updates and to say thanks.

Relationships

I was talking with a patient at our neighborhood open house, and she told me, "I never believed in love at first sight. That whole 'seeing someone across a crowded room' thing seemed sort of silly. I got my crowns just because it was practical, that's all. But then I'm at the gym and this really nice-looking guy is watching me, and he's not even trying to hide it, he's staring. Finally I just stare back, like, okay, you got something you want to tell me? And he just laughs, and then I laugh, and we're both smiling, and he comes over says, 'I'm sorry if I'm being obvious, but you have a beautiful smile.'

"Five months later, we're talking about the future. I'm a little giddy because it's moving so fast, but I'll tell you, I can't stop smiling." She introduced me to the young man, and he can't stop smiling either.

Happiness

I just performed a full mouth restoration for the most extraordinary patient I ever treated.

She's an eight-year-old girl who's been moved from foster home to foster home since she was a baby. No one every took good care of her, and by the time she got to me, her mouth was in pretty bad shape. She's a tough kid, though, and she was a great little patient for a full week of work. In fact, she barely said a word. I didn't know until afterwards that she's never seen a dentist at all.

When we were done, I gave her a hand mirror and asked her to take a look. She burst into tears. "What's wrong?" I asked her. She climbed up and hugged me and said, "I never saw my smile until now."

❖ ❖ ❖

The best stories are simple, impactful, urgent and, of course, true. They don't go into detail about technique.

They do put good effects up front. They also express some of that joy and satisfaction *you* feel when you do something life-changing—your Inner Smile. They tell me you understand how much good you can do, and that you seek that satisfaction throughout in your practice. Finally, they emphasize the patient as the hero, not the dentist, because the patient had the good sense, courage, and initiative to get assistance from precisely the person who could do him or her the most good.

How does this follow A→C→B? I'm seeing myself in that story. That's my life. That's the feeling I want. That's a miraculous change you helped make, and I want that too. I'm leaping ahead in the change I need to make, and now that I'm committed to being that new and better version of myself, I'm ready to ask you to help me do it.

❖ ❖ ❖

EIGHT: SCATTER RICH SMILES

If you're looking for timely, topical subjects to talk about when you communicate with your patients and potential patients, just check the newspapers. On any given day, you'll find items like these:

- Patients with diabetes who are otherwise healthy are filing discrimination suits against their employers, and employers in turn are firing or declining to hire people who require any special accommodations for their diabetes. And we're raising a generation of children who show pre-diabetic symptoms. (Do you discuss nutrition and bad eating habits with your patients, or do you simply fix the damage?)

- The link between inflammation and chronic, even fatal disease, is finally being understood by the medical press, and some reports have appeared in the popular media. The connection between diet, habits like smoking and drinking, and chronic inflammation seems increasingly credible, but under the continual assault of advertising about the very things that may underlie the problem it's hard for the average consumer to hear the news they need, and to understand just how many problems they're eating and drinking every day. (Do your patients ever get constructive advice about their lifestyles from you? Do they connect causes and effects when they come to you for pain relief or improvements to their appearance?)

- People with pending diagnoses about life-threatening illnesses are left waiting for answers to questions from doctors who are too busy, or just otherwise unavailable, to give them time. The wait only raises the level of stress for both parties, turning doctors and patients into adversaries when their mutual dependence is greatest. It might get worse when the patient is actually in the hospital, their life on the line. Their dignity is lifted from them as casually and indifferently as their temperatures are taken. As one recent story put it, "the doctor ignored her. He talked about carcinomas and circled her bed like a presenter at a lawnmower trade show, while his audience, half-dozen medical students in their 20's, stared at Ms. Duffy's naked body with detached curiosity." (Have you performed full-mouth exams and discussed what you found with your patients? Has that conversation ever helped them avoid an incident like this one?)

- About one-third of the American population is obese. (See the above. Have you treated patients for whom you can realistically anticipate illnesses and problems related to their eating habits?)
- A medical search firm cites U.S. Bureau of Labor Statistics estimating only 25 of the 50 states have an adequate number of dentists. In many areas, there is only one practicing dentist for 2,000 people.
- *The Nation* reported in January, 2008, that "According to Maryland Senator Ben Cardin's staff, dental decay is now the most common chronic childhood disease in the US, affecting 20% of children aged 2 to 4, 50% of those aged 6 to 8, and nearly 60% of fifteen year olds. It is five times more common than asthma among school age children, and nearly 40% of African-

American children have untreated tooth decay in their adult teeth. Improper hygiene can increase a child's adult risk of having low birth-weight babies, developing heart disease, or suffering a stroke. 80% of all dental problems are found in just 25% of children, primarily those from lower-income families."

- The National Center for Health Statistics reports that "Adult use of antidepressants almost tripled between 1988-1994 and 1999-2000. Ten percent of women 18 and older and 4% of men now take antidepressants. Prescriptions for nonsteroidal anti-inflammatory drugs, antidepressants, blood glucose/sugar regulators and cholesterol-lowering statin drugs, in particular, increased notably between 1996 and 2002." (If you could build more smiles for these people, would they be as inclined to seek their relief from drugs?)

❖ ❖ ❖

You read the papers too, I know, and you're busy people, and the concern I felt at the outset of writing this book remains as strong for me at end as it ever was, that I might only be telling you a great deal that you already know. I'll take that risk, because the dentists

I know were so supportive of my modest effort, and so generous with their feedback and comments, that I thought these few words might actually be valuable, and might remind you of a couple of other things I hope you know.

"I have learned never to underestimate the capacity of the human mind and body to regenerate," Norman Cousins said, *"even when the prospects seem most wretched."* Cousins had the advantages of urgency, wise counsel, and his own profound intellect and curiosity to help him survive. I, a typical patient in your chair, might have none of these. But my life is on the line when I'm with you, sometimes quite literally, and always in the sense that new possibilities for it are sitting beside me. And if I settle for some sad, compromised version of it instead of the one I might have, then my prospects are wretched enough indeed.

I hope you know how badly needed you are. I hope you know the difference you make. The difference between me as I am, and me as I might be, may be you.

❖ ❖ ❖

The source of a true smile is an awakened mind. That source is you, if you choose to be awake to everything you could be, and to help awaken me.

I met a dentist once who nearly quit his practice. The debt he'd incurred from his education and from opening his office was hard to handle, and he was wasting even more money on failed marketing efforts and fruitless continuing education. After several years in practice, he despaired over having made the wrong choice with his life, but the financial corner he was in cut off all his options. He had no choice except to work harder, which just made things feel worse.

Someone familiar stopped him on the street one day. The dentist vaguely recognized the man as a former patient, someone he hadn't seen in a long time. The man told him that he'd moved away to further his career and had recently returned. He described his terrific success in his job, and the new home he owned, and his happy marriage, and he smiled as he told the dentist, "I feel like I should thank you for all of it." Now the dentist recognized him. He knew those crowns.

The baffled dentist asked, "What do you mean?"

"I never understood what it meant to feel good about myself until I met you," the man said. "Until then, I felt like I was second-rate. I didn't realize how much I was hiding from people, how afraid I was to be seen. You worked on me for a couple of sessions and suddenly I looked like a different person. I *felt* like one. I started taking better care of myself. I paid attention to my health. My family life got better. My marriage got better. It helped my career. If I trace back everything good that's happened to me in the last few years, I think it started when you gave me a smile." The man shook the dentist's hand firmly and asked for an appointment card.

"I have to confess something," the dentist said. "I'm thinking of getting out of dentistry."

The man's grip tightened on the dentist's hand. "Oh no," he pleaded. "*No*, you can't do that. You must have a hundred patients like me—people whose lives you changed. People who need you." The man searched the dentist's eyes and asked, "Don't you understand how much good you do? Do you realize what you really do for a living?"

Whose story is that?

It's not just the patient's. It's your story, too, and so is every story of every patient who sits in your chair. Your life changes when you change my life, and every investment you make in me—or decline to make—creates a return in you. Your renewal of me, the joy, the health and the possibilities you create for me, must—they *must*—give you some measure of the same things. If you accept them, you improve with everyone you improve. If you seek only to fix, you seek only to be repaired. It's much too little for you to ask. You deserve more.

Do you realize what you really do—*all* of it—for a living?

There's a prayer in the Hindu spiritual tradition that belongs at the center of everything I'm asking you to keep in mind. You can forget everything I've tried to say here if you remember this and live it in your work:

Let my soul smile through my heart and my heart smile through my eyes, that I may scatter rich smiles in sad hearts.

Surely, it was an enlightened sage who expressed this, for only someone wise, generous and touched with grace could commit to such an ambitious, beautiful aspiration.

It must have been a dentist.

ACKNOWLEDGEMENTS

I am very grateful for the advice and suggestions of dental practitioners and industry experts from across the United States. Both their enthusiasm and their criticism were of invaluable help. They affirmed for me, when I still questioned it, that this book may find an audience and serve a purpose.

I am particularly indebted to Lynn D. Carlisle, D.D.S., whose Web site, www.spiritofcaring.com, is an inspirational, practical resource for dentists seeking to improve their practices and their lives. Dr. Carlisle was a rigorous mentor in the creation of this book. It might not have happened without him.

My deepest thanks go to:

Dr. Lee Brady, Miami, FL

Dr. William Brown, Leon, IA

Ms. Joan Forrest,
St. Petersburg, FL

Dr. Cory Foster,
Fort Collins, CO

Dr. Gerard R. LeDoux,
St. Charles, MO

Dr. Bill Lockard,
Oklahoma City, OK

Dr. Mark T. Murphy,
Rochester Hills, MI

Dr. Bruce Pettersen,
Plymouth, MA

Dr. Mike Robichaux,
Slidell, LA

Dr. Gary Sellers,
Lafayette, CO

Dr. Gregory Tarantola,
Miami, FL

Dr. Michael R. Lewis,
Rochester, NY

Ms. Deb Castillo,
Bigfork, MT

Dr. Nancy Burkhart,
Charlotte NC

Dr. Steve Ratcliff,
Key Biscayne, FL

Dr. Steven D. Wegner,
Omaha, NE

Dr. Richard A. Green,
Sanibel, FL

Dr. Paul A. Henny,
Roanoke, VA

Dr. Ronald G.
Presswood, Houston, TX

Ms. Mary Osborne,
Seattle, WA

Dr. Lino Suarez Jr.,
Coral Gables, FL

Dr. Jeffrey Watson,
Syracuse, NY

Dr. Abby Brodie,
Coral Springs, FL

Dr. Bruce Peltier,
Brisbane, CA

Mr. Michael Brodie,
Coral Springs, FL

Dr. Deborah Anders,
Black Mountain, NC

BIBLIOGRAPHY

Cousins, Norman. *Anatomy of an Illness as Perceived by the Patient.* New York: W. W. Norton & Company. 2005.

Ring, Malvin E., D.S.D., M.L.S., F.A.C.D. *Dentistry. An Illustrated History.* New York: Harry N. Abrams, Inc. 1985.

Thich Nhat Hanh. *From Peace Is Every Step: The Path of Mindfulness in Everyday Life,* Bantam reissue, 1992, ISBN 0-553-35139-7.

Williams, Guy. *The Age of Agony.* Chicago: Academy Chicago Publishers. 1996.

Wynbrandt, James. *The Excruciating History of Dentistry.* New York: St. Martin's Griffin. 2000.

Various articles listed at www.spiritofcaring.com.

The "Let my soul smile" quote is from Paramahansa Yogananda.

REFERENCES

1. "U.S. life expectancy still trails 30 countries". CNN.com/health. June 11, 2008. www.cnn.com/2008/HEALTH/06/11/life.expectancy.ap/index.html. Accessed August 29, 2008

2. "Health care spending in U.S. reached $1.6 trillion in 2002". *USA Today,* Health and Behavior, posted 1/8/2004. http://www.usatoday.com/news/health/2004-01-08-health-care_x.htm. Accessed October 3, 2008.

3. "U.S. Health Care Spending to Double by 2017, Report Predicts." By Steven Reinberg, HealthDay Reporter. February 26, 2008; *Washington Post,*

http://www.washingtonpost.com/wp-dyn/
content/article/2008/02/26/AR2008022601380.
html. Accessed October 3, 2008.

4. Harker, L.A., & Keltner, D. (2001). Expressions of positive emotion in women's college yearbook pictures and their relationship to personality and life outcomes across adulthood. *Journal of Personality and Social Psychology*, 80, 112-124.

5. Thich Nhat Hanh, *From Peace Is Every St*ep: The Path of Mindfulness in Everyday Life, Bantam reissue, 1992, ISBN 0-553-35139-7

How to Obtain this Book

Please visit www.amazon.com, www.fromthechair.com or www.booksurge.com for additional copies

ABOUT THE AUTHOR

David Clow's journalism has appeared in national, local, business and academic publications covering topics from news, features, and business issues to the obscure events behind America's successful lunar exploration. His corporate communications have served *Fortune* 100 market leaders in energy, telecommunications, software, and a range of other industries.

David is the writer of the documentary film series Understanding Cities, showing the historical evolution of Rome, Paris, London, American cities and the city of the future. He is co-author of *Six Lessons for Six Sons* (Harmony, 2006, Three Rivers, 2007), which *Ebony* called "An awe-inspiring story of fatherly love and dedication."

A graduate of the University of Pennsylvania, he is a member of the Authors Guild, the American Medical Writers Association and the National Association of Science Writers.